USMLE Step 2
Clinical Skills Triage

USMLE Step 2 Clinical Skills Triage

A Guide to Honing Clinical Skills

Kevin Schwechten, MD

Teaching Faculty and Staff Physician

Magnolia Regional Health Center
Magnolia Regional Health Center Residency Program
Corinth, Mississippi

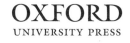

OXFORD
UNIVERSITY PRESS

2010

OXFORD
UNIVERSITY PRESS

Oxford University Press, Inc., publishes works that further
Oxford University's objective of excellence
in research, scholarship, and education.

Oxford New York
Auckland Cape Town Dar es Salaam Hong Kong Karachi
Kuala Lumpur Madrid Melbourne Mexico City Nairobi
New Delhi Shanghai Taipei Toronto

With offices in
Argentina Austria Brazil Chile Czech Republic France Greece
Guatemala Hungary Italy Japan Poland Portugal Singapore
South Korea Switzerland Thailand Turkey Ukraine Vietnam

Published by Oxford University Press, Inc.
198 Madison Avenue, New York, New York 10016

www.oup.com

Library of Congress Cataloging-in-Publication Data

Schwechten, Kevin.
USMLE step 2 clinical skills triage : a guide to honing clinical skills / Kevin Schwechten.
p. ; cm.
Includes index.
ISBN 978-0-19-539823-6
1. Clinical medicine—Examinations, questions, etc.   2. Clinical medicine—Case studies.
3. Physicians—Licenses—United States—Examinations—Study guides.
4. Medical history taking—Examinations, questions, etc.   5. Medical history taking—Case studies.
6. Diagnosis, Differential—Case studies.   7. Diagnosis, Differential—Examinations, questions, etc.   I. Title.
[DNLM: 1. Physical Examination—methods—Case Reports.   2. Physical Examination—methods—
Examination Questions.   3. Diagnosis, Differential—Case Reports.   4. Diagnosis, Differential—Examination
Questions.   5. Physician-Patient Relations—Case Reports.   6. Physician-Patient Relations—Examination
Questions. WB 18.2 S412u 2010]
RC58.S39 2010
616.0076—dc22
2009045015

ISBN: 978-0-19-539823-6

9 8 7 6 5 4 3 2 1

Printed in USA
on acid-free paper

To my amazing family: Dawn, my wife, whose support has meant everything, and to my children, Ariel and Tristan who gave me the great gifts of motivation, inspiration, and hope.

Also, to the soldiers, medics, and officers of the U.S. Army's 2–4 Infantry battalion, 10th Mountain Division (2008), who did a truly professional job in Iraq and made it possible for all of us to come home.

About the Author

Kevin Schwechten, born in Montana, earned his medical doctorate from Oregon Health & Science University in Portland, Oregon. He joined the U.S. Army during medical school and completed his Family Medicine residency at Martin Army Community Hospital in Fort Benning, Georgia. After training, he spent over a year as battalion surgeon in Baghdad, Iraq, where he cared for both soldiers and the Iraqi populace. Dr. Schwechten now lives, works, and teaches in Mississippi.

Contents

Section 1: Logistics of Step 2 Clinical Skills

Eligibility

Candidates for Step 2 CS must fulfill one of the following requirements to take the test:

- Be enrolled in or a graduate of a U.S. or Canadian medical school certified by the Liaison Committee of Medical Education (LCME) and have or be expected to receive an MD degree.

- Be enrolled in or a graduate of an osteopathic school certified by the American Osteopathic Association (AOA) and have or be expected to receive a DO degree.

- Be enrolled in or a graduate of a foreign medical school outside the United States or Canada certified by the Educational Commission for Foreign Medical Graduates (ECFMG).

Additional requirements or exceptions to requirements may be available in extenuating circumstances for those applicants in certain circumstances. These usually include MD/Ph.D. applicants and ECFMG candidates. Check the USMLE website (www.usmle.org) for these requirements.

Registration

Registration must be done through the websites for the appropriate candidate. U.S. and Canadian medical school students/applicants may go through the NBME site; international medical school graduates (IMGs) must go through the ECFMG site. These are: www.nbme.org and www.ecfmg.org, respectively. Both sites have an area to click on to be directed to a login that will give access to features such as:

- Application submission for the USMLE Step 2 CS.
- Request score documents.
- Print your scheduling permit.
- View the calendar of available test dates.
- Request an exam date.
- Change or edit exam date requests.
- Print various paper request forms.
- Print confirmation notices for the chosen test date.

After registration and fee payment, you will be issued a testing permit that gives a 12-month eligibility period during which you can take the test. The 12-month clock starts after the application is approved. Notice that a calendar of available tests dates is available online. This allows for scheduling based on the test center location and planning for the best time for you to take the exam. The strategy with scheduling is to pick the best date based on your own schedule, available transportation, available accommodations, and matching up with other professional or school schedules. Do not expect to "play the calendar" by requesting several dates. Only one date is allowed when scheduling is made, so be sure you can make that date (although this can be rescheduled if that date later becomes impossible to attend). Rescheduling will only be allowed within the 12-month eligibility period, and you will be charged an additional fee if rescheduling is requested within 14 days of a test date. If you miss your test date, for any reason, you will be allowed to reschedule but with a much higher rescheduling fee.

Calendar Scheduling Operates Under Several Rules:

- First come, first served. The sooner you request a date, the higher likelihood you'll receive the date you want.

- Scheduling, rescheduling, and opening of new calendar dates (based on demand at the particular center) all influence available dates. If at first a "must-have" date isn't available, make the second-most desirable date appointment, and check back for a change in availability. An e-mail function on the calendar scheduling website can also be used to notify you by e-mail when your desired date becomes available.

- If you cancel, make sure to reschedule at the same time. The system will not reschedule a cancelled appointment automatically.

Test Center Locations

There are five Clinical Skills Evaluation Center (CSEC) test centers located throughout the United States. These are:

1. CSEC Center—Atlanta

Two Crown Center

1745 Phoenix Boulevard

Suite 500, 5th Floor

Atlanta, GA 30349

2. CSEC Center—Chicago

First Midwest Bank Building, 6th Floor

8501 West Higgins Road, Suite 600

Chicago, IL 60631

3. CSEC Center—Houston

Amegy Bank Building, 7th Floor

400 North Sam Houston Parkway

Suite 700

Houston, TX 77060

4. CSEC Center—Los Angeles

Pacific Corporate Towers

100 North Sepulveda Boulevard, 13th Floor

El Segundo, CA 90245

5. CSEC Center—Philadelphia

Science Center

3624 Market Street, 3rd Floor

Philadelphia, PA 19104

Obviously, choosing the closest test center may provide greater familiarity and the least amount of cost; however, selection of center should be thought of as equal in every other way.

On Test Day

Arrive at least 30 minutes before the written arrival time on the scheduling confirmation. This is to ensure arrival in an unfamiliar testing center location and to allow for unexpected traffic (morning rush hour), and so forth. The testing session will be proceeded by a 30-minute orientation period, during which the test center may or may not allow entrance to late-comers. If the candidate arrives during this orientation period and admission is granted, they may be asked to sign a "Late Admission Form" stating they arrived late to the session. If this orientation period is missed and the candidate doesn't arrive in time, they will not be allowed into the test center and will have to reschedule with a late fee assessed.

Make sure to bring your scheduling permit, registration confirmation, an unenhanced **stethoscope,** a clean and empty **white laboratory coat**, and acceptable ID. Acceptable ID includes a passport, driver's license, national identity card (NIC), other government-issued ID card, or ECFMG identification card (if an IMG). The ID must have your picture (taken within the last 10 years) and signature. The name on the ID presented must match that on the scheduling permit exactly (with the exception of middle initial/name)—there will be *no* admittance for ID cards with maiden names, and so forth. At the test center, do not bring electronics, watches of any kind, or medical tools other than a stethoscope. You will be given a small locker, suitable for storage of small items like a purse or wallet, and provided access to a coat rack. If you desire, you may bring a small lunch (although it may not require refrigeration), although a lunch will be provided by the test center.

Breaks

There will be two breaks, the first consisting of 30 minutes, when a light lunch will be served, and a later 15-minute break. Unlike breaks given in Step 1 or Step 2 CK, these breaks can only be taken at the appointed time and not at the choosing of the candidate. During this time, bathroom breaks and lunch may be taken. Note that bathroom breaks won't be allowed at any other times. Smoking breaks or leaving the test center building for any reason during the appointed breaks is strictly forbidden.

Test Structure

The testing day consists of 12 patient encounters with "simulated patients," or SPs. Of these encounters, most will be scored, but there will also be one or two that are there solely for research purposes; of course, you will not know which ones are which. The test day lasts approximately 8 hours, including the breaks and initial orientation period.

Room Structure

The room is arranged to appear like the typical setting in which the encounter is occurring—that is, clinic exam room, hospital room, ER, and so forth. There will be an SP or telephone present. In encounters with an SP, there will either be a one-way glass partition or a closed circuit camera in which physician proctors are recording/observing the encounter. You should know both the physician-observers and the SP are grading your encounter.

When summoned to do so, you may approach the door and read the information posted on it about the case. This is called **"doorway information"** and includes the patient's name, chief complaint, vital signs, and instruction (which are usually the same between cases). Doorway information may also include pertinent lab studies previously ordered if this encounter is to be a follow-up, which may be the case. You should commit the patient's name to memory and process as much of the information as possible. Then, enter the room to start the patient encounter.

When entering, you should have your stethoscope and white lab coat as well as a provided clipboard with either blank paper or dry-erase board and pen in which to jot notes during the encounter. These notes may be used during the documentation period to remind you of pertinent details. When writing or reading notes during the patient encounter, it is typical to also make eye contact to ensure good communication with the SP.

When the patient encounter section of the case is complete (by hearing the announcement you'll know when this is, *see* below), you'll have an opportunity to document the encounter. Exit the room, where both a computer and a paper record will be available for this purpose. *Choose either the computer or paper method to document.* If the computer is chosen, there are assigned fields in which to fit the History, Physical Exam, Differential Diagnosis, and Work-up plan. The differential diagnosis and work-up plan are both limited to five options so don't expect to list every possibility or test you think might be occurring going on. If using the computer version of the patient encounter note, the computer automatically limits the number of characters available in each field, and when this number has been entered, no further typing will be recorded (the field will not accept new characters). On the right of the field, there will appear a scroll bar when the number of characters exceeds that in the field but is still less than that allowed. Scroll up and down to review entered text. Conversely, if the paper method is chosen, there will be fields available for the same. Do not write outside the thin line border around the paper's edge because these documents are scanned into digital format after the test, and whatever is written outside the border won't be captured by the scanner.

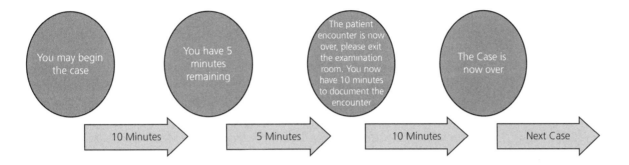

Announcements

Each case consists of a **15-minute patient encounter** and a **10-minute interval** for documentation. Within the 15 minutes of patient encounter interaction, the patient's history of present illness and other pertinent data about the chief complaint must be gathered and any questions answered. A focused physical exam must also be performed. Then the closure of the case with explanation of the differential diagnosis and work-up plan must be done. Needless to say, this is not much time for a complete interaction, thus your interaction should be focused on pertinent information-gathering and interaction. You will then have 10 minutes to document the encounter. Remember, re-entering the room is strictly forbidden under any circumstances, so don't exit the encounter unless you either are told to do so by an announcement or are absolutely sure you have all the information you need.

Scoring

The encounter is scored by the combination of several different components, as seen below. The SP scores the patient based mainly on encounter interactions and physical exam skills, whereas the physician-observers score mainly on technical correctness and documentation. Each subcomponent will be given a score, and the scores for each case are then tallied. The average of each component must add to a "passing" score to receive a "pass" for the whole exam.

Scores

The total score of the CS exam consists of averaging each score for all cases (except those used in research). Each case is scored based on three subcomponents: Integrated Clinical Encounter (ICE) score, Communication and Interpersonal Skills (CIS) score, and Spoken English Proficiency (SEP) score. The sub-subcomponents of each are as follows:

Integrated Clinical Encounter (ICE):

Data-gathering
- information collected by history taking and physical exam as seen by the SP.

Documentation
- completion of a patient note summarizing the patient encounter, differential diagnosis, and **initial** work-up plan.

Note that the data-gathering score is **generated by the SP** and is scored with the use of checklists. These checklists are developed by the physician committee's that create the test and are specific to the pertinent information to each case. The SP will not be going through the checklist during the encounter but will score you after you exit the room. The documentation component of the ICE will be scored by trained physician-raters and will also be done after the case has ended. Documentation is scored not only on how complete the details of the case are written down but also the accuracy of the differential diagnosis and appropriateness of the work-up plan. Keep in mind, in all the patient encounters, more than one diagnosis is possible, so don't try to find the one solution to the problem presented.

Communication and Interpersonal Skills (CIS):
Questioning skills:
- Use of open-ended questions, transitional statements, and facilitating statements.
- Avoid leading or multiple questions, repeating questions unless for clarification, medical/technical terms unless immediately defined, and interruptions when the patient is talking.
- Accurately summarizing information from the patient during the interview.

Information-sharing skills:
- Acknowledging patient concerns and clearly responding with information addressing the concern.
- Providing counseling when appropriate.
- Providing closure, including explanation of the next step in diagnosis/plan.

Professional manner and rapport:
- Asking about expectations, feelings, and concerns.
- Assessing support systems and impact of illness on the personal life.
- Showing consideration for patient comfort during the physical examination.
- Demonstrating attention to cleanliness through hand washing or use of gloves.
- Providing opportunity for the patient to express feelings/ concerns.
- Encouraging additional questions or discussion.
- Making empathetic remarks concerning patient issues/ concerns.
- Making the patient feel comfortable and respected during the encounter.

The CIS is **scored by the SP** and provides a global score based on their impressions of the CIS components. The patient encounter is broken down, and each component of the CIS is rated by the SP based on scales developed by the physician committee creators and is designed to provide an objective assessment of each component. However, this is the most subjective component of the overall score because the SP is allowed a certain amount of subjective impression to rate each component of the encounter. Thus, connecting with the SP on a personal level, or attempting to do so, is the root of this score.

Spoken English Proficiency (SEP):

- Clarity of spoken English communication within the context of the doctor–patient encounter (e.g., pronunciation, enunciation, word choice, and minimizing the need to repeat phrases).

The SEP portion of the score is **given by the SP** and is based on clarity and comprehension of the SP to understand what the candidate meant to say. This component should be the easiest for native English-speaking candidates but may represent somewhat of a barrier to non-English-speaking or non-proficient candidates.

Score Reporting

Candidates taking Step 2 CS are classified into groups based on when the exam was taken. A reporting period is then assigned to each group corresponding to when the score report will be available. The USMLE reserves the right to not report any score until the last day of the reporting period, although the majority of scores for a given period will be available on the first day of the reporting period. Reporting of scores can occur 4 to 12 weeks after the test was actually taken. A chart of the test periods and the corresponding reporting periods may be found at www.usmle.org or http://www.usmle.org/Examinations/step2/step2cs_reporting.html.

Section 2: USMLE Clinical Skills Strategy

Strategy

Putting it into Perspective

The Step 2 CS exam tests skills that are meant to be at the root of all physician–patient interactions. These skills are consistent with a patient-centered information-gathering period, synthesizing of information gathered, and the production a plan of action to address these concerns. These are skills all medical students should be working on during their medical education from the start. However, these don't always come naturally, especially in front of a patient that has the power to steer your medical career in a bad direction and a hidden physician lurking in an adjacent room. It's important to realize, however, you shouldn't be intimidated by these facts. The presence or absence of this evaluation shouldn't radically change what you do every time you interact with a patient—that is, your skills as you interact with a patient on the wards without anyone else there shouldn't be much different than that demonstrated on the test. This is a good thing. Thus, as corny as it sounds, you can hone your interaction skills with every patient you see, and everyone you see is an opportunity to study for this test.

A Word on Practice

Your patient interaction for Step 2 CS has been objectified as much as possible with rating scales and standardized exam findings. The point to these rating scales is to produce consistency across a broad range of test candidates in an attempt to compare each individual person to the next in a reproducible way. However, much ground may be covered by the candidate that is confident and forthright although not technically correct in every way. This is because of the inherent subjectivity of this style of test. No matter what the rating scale used to score an interaction, initial impression by the SP means a lot, especially when giving the CIS score (*see* Section on Scoring). Thus, it's important you project a confident and professional demeanor during the interaction with the SP. This confident manner comes naturally to some and with great difficulty to others. However, the saving grace for all candidates is the fact that your manner of interaction improves with practice. The more patients you see, the more the interaction cues and turning points become expected and clear. After repetition hones these skills, more brain energy can be spent on thinking about the differential diagnosis and work-up plans as you're speaking with the patient. Remember, the best way to study for this exam is practice with real patients. Develop your rapport, develop your confidence, and once you have these down, this test will become much easier.

The Patient Encounter Interview

Doorway Information

---

1. Opening Scenario

Mark Picks, a 73-year-old male presents to the physician's office with complaints of bloody diarrhea for the last week.

2. Vital Signs

BP: 120/82 mmHg

Temp: 98.0° F (36.7° C)

HR: 66/minute, regular

RR: 12/minute

3. Examinee Tasks

1. Obtain a focused history.

2. Perform a relevant physical examination. (Do not perform breast, pelvic/genital, or rectal examination.)

3. Discuss your initial diagnostic impression and your work-up plan.

4. After leaving the room, complete your patient note on the given form.

Initial Impressions

Things to Memorize on the Doorway Information:

- The patient's name, which you'll use directly after entering the room.
- The patient's age.
- The patient's chief complaint and time-course, if available.
- Any lab information presented.

Check the vital signs for abnormalities and memorize any that are not within the normal limits. Always ask yourself "Are the vital signs stable?"

Check the examinee tasks for instructions that vary from other doorway information. The vast majority won't differ, although at least skimming these for changes may prove well worth it.

Knock on the door gently, and enter.

> Give yourself time to process the doorway information. A few extra seconds here may make a big difference in the room.

Signposts

Signposts are statements or phrases that let the SP know where you're going with the conversation. These may be a statement such as "I understand you've been having periods of vomiting. Please tell me more about it," which tells the patient you know that their problem is vomiting and you'd like to talk about that instead of some other accompanying symptom they might have. Or simply stating "I'd like to do a physical exam now. Would you please remove your shoes for me?" tells the patient your intent is to move on to the physical part of the interaction, and it will start with their feet. These are simple statements that prepare the patient for what you're expecting to do so the transition is more comfortable.

The two main areas for the use of signposts are in the beginning of the interaction, during the introduction and at the transition of the history-taking and physical exam portions. However, signposting may also be used to introduce a sensitive style of questions within the interview, such as sexual history taking or depression questioning. As well, at the end of the physical exam and introduction to the counseling portion, you may want to signpost your thoughts of the encounter and the work-up plan. In this case, the signpost statement can be used as the introduction to the counseling, such as "Ok, Mr Jones, after hearing about your symptoms and doing the physical exam, I'm going to go over what I think might be wrong and what we can do to further figure it out." This is a good indication of your intent to transition.

Beginning the Interview

When you enter the room, notice what setting is portrayed. A hospital or ER setting dictates a different interview style than a clinic visit.

Introduce yourself by formal name, Dr. Soandso, and address the patient by their formal name, Mr./Ms. Smith. Do not address them using their first name! Then signpost the interview using a question about their chief complaint, but make sure you leave the question open-ended. That is, state "I understand your joints have been hurting. Please tell me more about this," rather than "I understand you've been having joint pain. Is that correct?"

Interview Body

The interview should then be conducted very much like an **"inquisitive conversation."** That is, respond to the patient's complaints appropriately and not to solely mine for data, which may come off cold. Otherwise, interview styles will vary, but all should be guided by the principle of obtaining information in a patient-friendly manner.

See below for elements that should be utilized in the interview body:

Element of interview	Approach and examples
Pain can be explored by using the mnemonic: OPQRST	O-onset P-Provoking factors Q-Quality/quantity on scale of 0–10 R-Radiation S-Symptoms associated with the pain T-timing during the day or night
Signpost difficult lines of questioning	Sexual history Depression or abuse
Transition statements of empathy (TSEs)	"I'd feel the same way if I were you…" "That must've been hard to deal with at the time…"

If the patient has an immediate concern in the beginning of the interview "On-demand signposting"	Address the concern by stating that you'd also like to find the answer to their question and that the best way to do this is to continue with the interview and physical exam. Explain the normal format of the encounter (history-taking, then physical exam) so the patient knows what to expect.
Clarification of previously discussed issues	When the patient steers the interview away from a point you'd like clarified, initially, allow them to do so. However, after the pressing issue is explored, return to the previous point for clarification questions.
When a patient admits to significant alcohol use	Rule of Thumb for CAGE questions: Ask questions if: >2 drinks/day for men >1 drink/day for women
	CAGE questions: C—"Have you ever tried to **C**ut down?" A—"Have you ever felt **A**nnoyed by those around you asking about your drinking?" G—"Have you ever felt **G**uilty because of your drinking?" E—"Have you ever had an '**E**ye opener' or a drink in the morning to get you going?"

Physical Exam

Signpost the transition to physical exam. You should start by explaining what initial system you are going to evaluate. Statements such as "Please let me begin by looking inside your ear canals" work well. However, explaining the transition between each individual system is not necessary.

When performing a physical on the SP, do not perform the "forbidden" exams.

Forbidden exams
Female breast
Genitals
Inguinal hernia (although inguinal node exam is permissible)
Corneal reflex
Rectum/anus
Throat swabs

Before you uncover each area for exam, ask permission or simply ask the patient to uncover that part of their body for you.

Several rules to abide by are:
- Don't perform painful maneuvers more than once.
- Accept simulated responses as real.
- If one of the "forbidden" exams is necessary, write it on the work-up plan.
- Don't press too hard on the patient in the expectation of a better response.
- On female patients wearing bras, it is permissible and expected to ask them to move them for an adequate exam.

A Word on Focus

When performing the physical exam in the pertinent systems, it's not always necessary to perform every possible aspect of the exam to attain an adequate amount of information for the patient. That is, a "shotgun" approach of evaluating all aspects of what can be evaluated often yields much information that isn't useful in the ultimate diagnosis and causes a needless time delay. Rather, having heard the history from the patient, your approach should be to perform a focused physical exam with particular emphasis on those aspects that may support or refute your working differential diagnosis. For example, obtaining a measurement for diaphragmatic excursion on a patient you suspect as having tuberculosis may not be helpful enough to spend the extra time on. The scoring SP and the physician evaluators take into account the time constraint of this test, and thus, a **pertinent and focused physical exam is of high value.**

Maneuvers to Show

When performing the physical exam, rarely will the SP actually have a real finding. Most findings are simulated. This is done with the SP acting or with makeup over the affected part. However, when doing the physical, it's often easy to get wrapped up in thought and not explain what it is you're doing. Thus, you should definitely show and/or describe that you're performing a particular exam. For example, if performing an abdominal exam and observing the patient's abdomen, an out-loud statement of "Your abdomen doesn't look distended, and there doesn't appear to be any bruising" may earn valuable points as an alternative to simply staring at their abdomen for a few seconds.

Information-Gathering During the Physical Exam

Information can continue to be obtained while doing the physical to both clarify positive findings and to save time on the overall encounter. Questions such as "Has this spot always been this tender?" may help to clarify previously discussed points.

Closure

The closure of the case should be done knowing that this is basically your time to talk the most. Certainly the patient should feel free to interrupt and ask questions, but this is also your time to verbally give your interpretations and work-up plan. Thus, elements should be included to help the patient understand what you're thinking and to know what to expect. It is vitally important that long, technical language be left out of this section unless immediately and totally explained.

Strategy for Closure

The best strategy is to explain at least the top two diagnoses on your differential and go into more depth about the concerns and testing you plan to obtain. During the explanation of these diagnoses, explain to the patient the elements in the history and physical exam that lead you to that conclusion. For example, if a patient has what you think is GERD, explain that you think this is so because of their recurrence of symptoms with spicy foods, symptoms when lying down after eating, burning sensation in their chest, acidic taste in their mouth after big meals, and the reproduction of pain on palpation of their epigastrum. Taking elements from the history and physical exam will not only help the patient understand your conclusion but can pre-empt any clarification questions they have at this stage, as time is usually tight when at the conclusion.

When explaining the differential diagnosis, some diagnoses may require more counseling than others. If any kind of cancer is thought likely, a full explanation should be given. Especially with words such as "cancer," patients and SPs get visions of death or major impairment. Hence the need for complete explanation that you won't be able to tell them today that they do or don't have cancer but that further testing will help you decide.

Explanation of testing is also of importance as this is the next step the patient can focus on. Often, the diagnosis won't be certain and testing is needed; the patient will feel much more comfortable with your care if they know exactly what the tests are for and what they will tell you once the results come back. Good explanation of the tests and where it leads in the path to definitive diagnosis will leave the patient with a clear path of focus about the future.

Statement of Ending

When finally ending the patient encounter, an exit strategy is needed. Because, in these cases, a definitive diagnosis and plan to treat is not expected to be given, a statement to transition to further work-up may be used. That is, a statement of arrangement of the previously discussed tests can be useful to end the encounter. For example, "I'd like to step out now to arrange your blood samples with my nurse" is much better than "The encounter is over, so I'm going to leave now." At this point, time is typically short and the SP will understand you're trying to exit the room; however, you'll get credit for making a good excuse to leave rather than leaving under awkward circumstances.

Final Sentence

In the final sentence you should leave the encounter open-ended and friendly and also thank the SP for their time. This statement should be memorized and leave the SP with a confident and openly positive impression as the last thing they remember. The statement "Is there any other aspect of your health care we haven't already discussed? Ok then, thank you." is very effective and functions well to give the SP a final opportunity to talk about anything you might have missed (if they would want to) and politely concludes the encounter.

Documentation

Notes During the Patient Encounter

During the patient encounter, you will be provided with either a blank piece of paper or a dry-erase board and pen. It's expected that while conducting the history and physical exam you write down notes to keep track of details that are presented throughout the encounter. These notes may become very valuable in a complicated case to refer to in the closure section or when documenting the case. Keep in mind, after documentation is complete, these notes will be destroyed or erased.

A Suggestion for Notes

It's recommended you use your notes as a "working" differential diagnoses list as well as a detail-recording device. That is, in the margin of the notes, you can list possible diagnoses that come to mind during the encounter. If you think of one diagnosis during the encounter, add it to the list; if another you previously thought might be possible is disproven, cross it off. This allows for a smooth and swift transition to closure at the end of the case.

Notes	Ddx
-CC: Knee pain for three days -Hurts in the anterior knee -Worse with running or jumping -No swelling or redness -Hurts at night	Bursitis ~~Osgood-Schlatter's~~ ACL tear Meniscus tear ~~Septic joint~~ Osteoarthritis Rheumatoid arthritis

Formal Documentation

After the patient encounter is over, 10 minutes is allotted to document what you have just gone through. This is expected to be a focused note and provide a trained physician evaluator a sample of what should be written for the given encounter. It bears repeating that this note is not expected to be a verbose and completely accurate portrayal of what occurred with the SP; it's meant to be a note consistent with the encounter. Abbreviations may be used, but you should only use those approved and on the official "abbreviation list," which will be immediately available to you during your documentation period (usually taped to the wall on the desk). This list is available at the USMLE website and should be looked over before the exam. Some exceptions to the listed abbreviations are seen on the sample notes available for download from the USMLE website. There are several shorthand abbreviations used in those notes that are very common and considered legal. However, a word of warning: be very certain the abbreviations you use are either on the abbreviation list or are VERY COMMON to all shorthand styles seen in medicine.

Instructions Given on the Patient Note

History: Include significant positives and negatives from history of present illness. Past medical history, review of system(s), social history, and family history.

Physical Exam: Indicate only pertinent positive and negative findings related to the patient's chief complaint.

Format

There will be two formats available to you to choose from when documenting the patient encounter: a paper, handwritten note or a computerized note. The handwritten version may be done in several styles that are given as examples by the USMLE committee. You should familiarize yourself with both styles before the test.

The first style involves a paragraph version where the history of present illness is written using abbreviations in a paragraph narrative. Sentences are succinct and short, and abbreviations are plentiful. The second style is to use bullets for pertinent information and different aspects of the history. Physical exam in either style consists of sections labeled by system, and each briefly explains pertinent positives or negatives. In the computerized documentation format, comparable room for typing is provided, although a paragraph style of writing is assumed. In this format, the field is limited to a certain number of characters, after which no further typing will be recorded. Thus, your note should be shorter than this limit. However, keep in mind that this limit is somewhat greater than expected when looking at the field itself, which necessitates a scroll bar on the right side to appear when the typing goes beyond what is immediately visible.

When documenting your findings, either in the history or the physical exam section, remember to only write the significant positive and negative findings. Minute details of the history or insignificant physical exam findings may not need to be documented.

For phone encounters or those where the parent or guardian is the only person present when describing a child, a physical exam can't be done, and the physical exam section can be left blank.

Differential Diagnosis

This section allows five and only five diagnoses to be given. These diagnoses should be ordered from the most likely disease (1) to the least likely (5). Do not use symptoms as diagnoses unless there is clearly no other medical term for the condition. For example, use "cholecystitis" instead of "right upper quadrant pain." It's also worth noting that if you don't think there are five diagnoses that are possible, you don't have to fill all five places. You should use the differential diagnosis section as a list of possibilities that need further exploration using the work-up plan you develop in the next section. Keep in mind; they're a list of possibilities, not a list of answers to a question that has a specific solution.

Instructions Given on Patient Note

Differential diagnoses: In order of likelihood (with 1 being the most likely), list up to 5 potential or possible diagnoses for this patient's presentation (in many cases, fewer than 5 diagnoses are likely):

Diagnostic Work-up

This section also has five, and only five, possible investigational options that can be ordered. The diagnostic plan can include almost anything from a "forbidden" exam to blood tests, to imaging, to diagnostic procedures. However, DO NOT expect to be able to place other options here, such as consultations, exams, questions you should have performed/asked but didn't, or treatment options. A "trial of treatment" will *not* be considered a work-up plan option. These tests are meant to prove/disprove the diagnoses you placed in the differential diagnosis section. Because these options are blank, almost any test, imaging choice, or diagnostic procedure is fair game. If after the case you believe there are no diagnostic studies needed for the work-up plan, write "no studies indicated" rather than leaving this section blank.

Instructions Given for Diagnostic Work-up

List immediate plans (up to 5) for further diagnostic work-up.

It should also be noted that the diagnostic work-up should consist of the next step in diagnosis of the patient, not definitive testing to make a definite diagnosis. For example, it's more appropriate to order an ECG on a patient before ordering a cardiac catheterization, thus, a cardiac catheter should not be on the work-up plan.

Abbreviations in Lab Tests

When entering lab tests in the diagnostic work-up section, it is permissible to list common tests, such as "CBC" instead of "WBCs, Hct, Hgb, and Platelets." Although if there is any doubt on what is included in a certain test, parentheses may be used to include those tests (e.g., "BMP" may be written as "BMP [Na, K, Cl, HCO3, BUN, Creat, Glu]").

1   Vision Loss

1. Opening Scenario

Elmer Michaelson, a 71-year-old male presents to the physician's office with complaints of worsening vision.

2. Vital Signs

BP: 152/94 mmHg

Temp: 97.9° F (36.6° C)

HR: 70/minute, regular

RR: 12/minute

3. Examinee Tasks

1. Obtain a focused history

2. Perform a relevant physical examination. (Do not perform breast, pelvic/genital, or rectal examination.)

3. Discuss your initial diagnostic impression and your work-up plan.

4. After leaving the room, complete your patient note on the given form.

Are the Vital Signs Stable?

Subjective

Knock; enter. Introduce yourself and place the first signpost.

"Hi, Mr. Michaelson, I'm Dr. Klein, I'm glad to see you today. I understand you've come in because of some recent vision changes. Please tell me more about this."

"Hi Dr. Klein. Yeah, I've come in for my **vision**. I'm getting older and my eyes just aren't what they used to be, you know? My **vision has been getting worse for years**. As you can see, I wear **bifocals**, I have for years, but I feel like it's just **getting worse**. I have a tough time seeing anything unless I look straight at it and even then sometimes it's hard to make out if it's too far away. Then at night, it's really hard to see almost anything. I mean, I can get around, but it's just hard."

"Ok, sir, how long would you say it has been since your vision has really started to get worse?"

"It's been a **few years**. I've worn these glasses for many years, now. I mean, maybe **30**, my eye doctor says I'm **near-sighted**. So, I got the bifocals about 10 or 15 years ago. But lately it's been worse than just having to watch the news up close or even far away; it's been **hard to see**."

"When you say 'It's hard to see,' is it hard to see out in the peripheral, or edges of your vision, or is it harder when you look right at something?"

"It seems like **both are worse**. I don't see much out in the edges. That is, when I try to look at something, I have to look right at it, like when I'm watching TV. My grandkids are always running around, and half the time I can't see when they come from the side to climb on my lap. That's not too big a problem, but I know I used to be able to, sort of, tell things like that."

"Yeah, I can see how that would be hard to adjust to. When you look right at an object, or perhaps you're reading, are the words in focus?"

Age-related tendency to hold objects further away is a hallmark of presbyopia.

"Yeah, sometimes I have to **hold the paper kind of far away**, though. I think that's my age, but eventually I can see it. I don't read the paper much anymore because the print is so darn small. My wife got me a reading glass, you know, a **magnifier**? But I don't like using that thing."

"Has this vision problem stopped you from reading?"

Patients may express embarrassment with use of assistive devices. It's important to encourage them to look at the bigger picture of health benefits to get over this barrier.

"I guess so. I just **don't want to feel like people are watching me** try to read. I feel ridiculous with that magnifier staring at a book or paper."

"I'm sorry to hear that, although I can understand why you wouldn't want to use that magnifier. I'll do my best to find the cause of what's going on, but please allow me to encourage you to use those devices if it helps you read."

"Ok, doc, whatever you can do."

"Alright. You've had those glasses for a long time. I know you said you got your bifocals a while ago as well. Have you been seen by an optometrist or ophthalmologist since then?"

Recommendations are for yearly ophthalmologic checks for diabetics.

"Oh yes. I usually go **every couple of years** to get checked out. It's been a couple of years since the last check. Actually, maybe about **3 years**, now that you mention it. I have **diabetes**, too, so my regular doctor has me go see an eye doctor every now and then."

"Has that eye doctor ever said you have an eye disease, or have you ever had eye surgery?"

"**No**, never. He just says I should come back the next time."

"Ok. So I can understand today's problem better, do you feel that this lack of vision affects both eyes the same or is one worse than the other?"

"Both are the same. I haven't noticed a difference."

"Ok. Along with this change of vision have you had any eye pain or headaches?"

"**No**, not at all. I'm fine as far as that."

"I know you mentioned you have diabetes. Do you take insulin?"

"Oh, **yeah**. I take insulin and do my shots all the time. I can't wait for somebody to figure out a way to test blood sugar without sticking my finger. I'd rather not give myself shots in the belly either but those **finger sticks are what hurt**."

"Yeah, they sure do. For right now, though, that's the only way to be really sure of what your blood sugar is. Are you testing yourself regularly?"

"Yeah, I test **sometimes**. When I get sick, especially. I know my insulin regimen."

"How often do you test yourself?"

"About **twice a week**, maybe. I know how much insulin to take so I try not to test my fingers too much."

"Do you remember about how high your sugar levels are?"

"It depends but I'd say **120 to about 170**. If it's high, I'll give a little extra that day."

"Do you then go back and check to make sure your level came down?"

"Sometimes; **I hate pricking myself**. I've done it this way a long time and I'm not dead yet."

"That's true. I want to make sure you're around a long time, too. How long has it been that you've seen the doctor for your diabetes?"

"About **3 years or so**. I call him and get refills for my medicines, though. Other than this vision problem, everything's been fine."

"Do you keep a blood sugar log of your readings?"

"**Yup**."

"Did you bring your log today?"

"**Nah**, I don't usually carry it around. Not today."

"Ok. Can I ask what other diseases you see the doctor for?"

"Sure, I have **high blood pressure**; I have **stomach problems** sometimes, and **high cholesterol**. I take medicines for these. Too many if you ask me."

"Ok. Can you tell me what medicines?"

"Sure, I have a list right here [as he finds a piece of paper in his wallet]. My blood pressure medicines are called **benazepril** and **metoprolol**. I take **atorvastatin** for that high cholesterol, and my **insulin**. There's another one called **rabeprazole** that I take for my belly. Then I have some **antacids** that I take because it helps my indigestion. My doctor also tells me it's good for my bones, too."

"Great. Those help me understand your case a little more. How much insulin do you take?"

"Its **regular insulin** twice a day; **20 in the morning and 20 at night**. Then I take another kind called **glargine, 15 units**, at night."

"Alright. Have you seen the doctor for any other diseases in your life? Or have you ever spent the night in the hospital?"

"Yeah, over the years I've seen the doctor for a lot of things. I had an operation on my belly to **remove my gallbladder** about 5 years ago. I had a **hernia** after that in one of the spots they operated on. I had a **fall** 4 years

The patient likely will not openly confess to not controlling their diabetes tightly. Specific questions should be asked.

It's important to assure the patient your goals and theirs are the same.

If time allows in diabetic patients, always obtain the patient's insulin regimen and average blood sugar readings.

ago, and he said I nearly broke a hip! Let's see…I also had a **car accident** a long time ago, probably 15 years ago that landed me in the hospital for a **broken leg** and a **separated shoulder**. They operated on my leg at the time. That's about it."

"Is that all the surgeries in your life?"

"Well, I had my **tonsils** out when I was a kid. They did that back then, you know. I also had a **hemorrhoid** about 5 years ago, too. That's it, though."

"Ok. Do you smoke or use tobacco?"

"**Nope**, I've never done that. I don't like it, never have."

"Do you drink alcohol?"

"I **don't anymore**. I used to when I was younger. I never had a problem, but that's just what I did. Wasn't much, though."

"Ok. Do you have any allergies to anything?"

"**Nah**."

"Are there any major diseases in your family I should know about?"

"My daughter's got **diabetes**, too. Her's is the other kind though. All she has to do is take pills. Um, my **brother** died a year ago from a **heart attack**; Andy was 75 years old. Nothing else."

"Do you live with anyone?"

"Oh sure—my wife, Selma. We've been married 49 years. She's got diabetes and high blood pressure too. She's out shopping now, you know."

Signpost for the Physical Exam

"Ok, I'd like to do a physical exam now, if you don't mind. Just let me **wash my hands**. First I'd like to take a look at your eyes…"

Objective

Points for Every Exam:

- Wash hands.
- Comment on vital signs, even if normal.
- Tell the patient where you are going to examine and what to disrobe.
- Do not repeat painful maneuvers.

Physical Exam:

Perform a focused physical, by system, from the head down.

System	Exam elements	Findings in this patient
HEENT	Test the limits of peripheral vision. Test extra-ocular muscle movement. Use a Snellen eye chart to determine visual acuity with glasses on. Examine pupil reactivity and comment on external ocular abnormities. Full visual acuity is not needed in this setting.	PERRLA, extra-ocular muscles intact. Vision 20/30 bilaterally based on aided Snellen eye chart testing.
Retina	Use an ophthalmoscope to examine both retinas. Change focus to examine the anterior chamber/lens, and then focus on the retina. Note optic disc ratios and any abnormalities such as "cotton wool" spots or "dot-blot" hemorrhages.	Normal appearing retina. Normal approximate cup/disc ratio. No vessel abnormalities.

Continue to gather information as you do the physical exam. Comment aloud on any real or simulated abnormalities.

Example: *"I'm going to hold up my fingers up and slowly bring them toward the center of your vision, please tell me when you see them [while covering one eye]."*

Example: *"I know this light can be bright and this exam is uncomfortable because of that. Please bear with me, though, because it's really important that I see the back of your eye clearly."*

End of Case

End by explaining you have several ideas of what could be wrong and could cause these symptoms. Tell the patient the first two diagnoses on your differential list and the major tests you'd now like to perform.

Example: *"Mr. Michaelson, there are several possibilities that might explain your vision loss. Unfortunately, there are several reasons you might experience this because you have diabetes, high blood pressure, and are a little older; these are risk factors. All of those factors can contribute to diseases that affect vision. Glaucoma is one disease that may be at work here and results from high pressure in your eyes. There is a fairly simple way to determine the pressure in your eyes and that is by a machine that quickly blows a small puff of air onto the eye itself. It determines the pressure by how the eye responds, and the test only takes a quick moment to complete, I'd like to do that today. Another possibility is that you're experiencing something called diabetic retinopathy, which causes certain changes and problems to the back of the eye from long-term uncontrolled diabetes. For these and a few other possibilities, I'd like to do some specialized eye testing on you. Some of these tests will involve me placing drops in your eyes to dilate the pupils; this is mainly to get a better look at the back of your eyes. This will make you sensitive to bright lights for a few hours after the exam, but it really is the best way for me to do the exam. I'd like to do these tests today, if you don't mind. If there is anything I see on this exam, then I'll be asking you to go to a special eye doctor for another check. Because you're diabetic, it's a good idea to go to one anyway and be evaluated for eye problems like you used to. Please allow me to step out and arrange this with my nurse.*
Before I go, is there any other aspect of your health care we haven't already discussed? Ok then, thank you."

PATIENT NOTE

History: Include significant positives and negatives from history of present illness, past medical history, review of system(s), social history, and family history.

HPI: 71 y/o male with gradual, painless vision loss over the last 3 years. Symptoms involve both peripheral vision and central vision of both eyes. The pt wears bifocal glasses regularly but has noticed visual acuity declining when watching TV or reading. PMH is pertinent for likely uncontrolled diabetes secondary to not checking finger sticks often enough, although this is unproven. Reported average FSBS 120-170. No diabetic eye exam x 3 years.

PMH: Hypertension, hyperlipidemia, GERD.

PSH: Fractured leg, hernia, cholecystectomy, shoulder injury, tonsillectomy.

Tobacco: Denies.

EtOH: Denies.

Meds: metoprolol, benazepril, atorvastatin, rabeprazol, occasional antacids. Insulin regimen: Regular 20 units qAM, qPM, Glargine 15 units qhs.

FamH: Daughter-NIDDM, brother-deceased from MI.

Physical Examination: Indicate only pertinent positive and negative findings related to the patient's chief complaint.

VS Stable. BP 152/94 noted.

HEENT: Eyes: PERLA, extraocular muscles intact. Visual acuity 20/30 bilaterally corrected.

Retina: Undilated exam: Normal retina without signs of edema, vessel abnormalities, or blurring of the optic disc. Suboptimal exam resulting from undilated state.

Differential Diagnosis: In order of likelihood (with 1 being the most likely), list up to 5 potential or possible diagnoses for this patient's presentation (in many cases, fewer than 5 diagnoses are likely)	Diagnostic Work-up: List immediate plans (up to 5) for further diagnostic work-up
1. Diabetic retinopathy	1. Dilated eye exam
2. Glaucoma	2. Tonometry
3. Macular degeneration	3. Goldmann perimetry testing
4. Cataracts	4. Amsler chart testing
5. Presbyopia	5. Hemoglobin A1c

2   Red Eye

---

1. Opening Scenario

Genevieve Eathe, a 19-year-old female, presents to the physician's office with complaints of a red and irritated eye.

2. Vital Signs

BP: 135/82 mmHg

Temp: 98.8° F (37.1° C)

HR: 72/minute, regular

RR: 12/minute

3. Examinee Tasks

1. Obtain a focused history.

2. Perform a relevant physical examination. (Do not perform breast, pelvic/genital, or rectal examination.)

3. Discuss your initial diagnostic impression and your work-up plan.

4. After leaving the room, complete your patient note on the given form.

Are the Vital Signs Stable?

Subjective

Knock; enter. Introduce yourself, and place the first signpost.

"Hi Ms. Eathe, I'm Dr. Sanchez, nice to meet you today. I understand you have a red, irritated eye, is that correct? Please tell me about it."

"Hi Dr. Sanchez. Yeah, my **eye's hurt** now for a week. It's red and hurts when **I'm in a bright room or outside**, and my **vision's blurry** almost all the time. Like I said, it's been a week or so, but it's **gotten worse** since it came on. The pain is constant now and the lights bother me much more. I think its 'pink eye.'"

"Ok. It sounds like it's pretty hard to deal with. I understand that your eye hurts, especially with bright environments, and you have blurring of your

> Interject "transition statements of empathy" throughout the interview when the patient seems to complain of their illness. This projects a feeling of caring and understanding.

vision. And that these symptoms have gotten worse over the last week. Are there any other symptoms in addition to this?"

"Yeah, my **eye tears a lot**, too. I mean a lot. I'm always using a tissue to wipe away the tears. I'm in college and I try to go to lecture and stuff, but I think everyone thinks I have 'pink eye.' It's embarrassing. It seems like they want to stay away from me. Is that what it is?"

"Well, 'pink eye,' or 'conjunctivitis,' is one of the possibilities. I'll have to get the full story from you, and then do a good exam before I can tell. Sometimes these diagnoses require some testing, but I can't tell that until I get the full story. Either way, I'm here to help. Do you mind if I ask a few questions before I take a look?"

> When a patient is intent on a specific diagnosis, briefly discuss it but state emphatically that more information is needed, then move on.

"No, **that's fine**."

"Are there any other symptoms, such as areas of vision loss you've noticed?"

"**No**, that's about it."

"Ok, when this first started, was there an initial injury or event that might have lead to it?"

"Well, so I'm on my dorm softball team, and we **played a game outside** right before this started. It was fine. A little windy that day, but I didn't get hit with the ball or have any problems, ya know. Then when I went inside was the first time I kind of thought, 'Jeez, my eye kind of hurts.' It looked a little pink, you know, when I looked in the mirror, but it wasn't too bad. So I went to bed and it was fine. The next morning when I woke up it was watering a lot. Then all day that day it was sore and watering and stuff. I just thought it would go away, because I've had 'pink eye' before and it just takes a while for it to go away, but this hasn't, so I thought I should come in."

"Ok. It has been a while since this started, hasn't it? When did the blurring of your vision start?"

"It was about that **second day**. It didn't really start out very bad. More like it was just the **tears** that were hard to look through, but sometime after that it was kind of blurry. Now when I close my good eye, it's definitely **blurry**."

> In all cases of conjunctivitis, ask about contact lens wear.

"Can you see out of it at all or are there any parts of your vision that are missing?"

"Yeah, I can see, but it's just **blurry**. There's no blind spots, just **blurriness**."

"Do you wear contact lenses or glasses?"

"**No**, I don't need them."

"Ok. You said the pain started after the softball game and has gotten worse. On a scale of 0 to 10, 10 being the worst pain imaginable, where would you rate this pain?"

"Well, maybe a **5** or so. I mean, it's there, but it's not killing me or anything."

"Do you feel the pain anywhere else—I mean, how about in your eyelid or around your eye?"

"**Not really**."

"How would you describe the pain? Is it a burning sensation or a dull ache or something else?"

"It's sort of **sore**, kind of like an **ache**. Almost like I got hit there or something. It's hard to describe."

"Have you gotten hit in the eye with anything?"

"**No**, nothing."

"Do you feel the sensation that something may be in the eye itself?"

"It **felt like that in the beginning**. I looked and had my friends look. Then it started getting sore, sort of, and that feeling went away. It's more sore now. It was only the first night that I thought something might be in there. I think I was wrong, though."

"Has your other eye been affected in any way? Any of the same or different symptoms?"

"**No**, my other eye's fine. No problems."

"Alright, to go back to the symptom of watering in your eye, does it water at night as well?"

"**Yeah**, I wake up with these crusts on it. It's like goop in the side of my eye, you know, but it's a lot."

"Has anything made the pain worse or better?"

"No, not really. **Turning off the lights** is about the only thing that helps. The **light hurts it** and has stopped me from going to class the last few days. It just hurts."

"Have you had any other symptoms with this such as fever?"

"**No**, nothing else."

"How about recent illnesses like a cold or stomach problem?"

"**Nope**."

"Have you ever had other problems in your past medical history that you saw a doctor for?"

"I used to have something called **rheumatoid arthritis** for kids. I had pain in my knees and elbows, and my pediatrician said it was arthritis. My mom took me to some specialists when I was young. I **haven't had a flare-up** of that in a quite a **few years**, though. I think I out grew it. When I was a **baby,** my mom also says I almost died from **meningitis**. It was when I was really young—just a baby—so I don't know. She calls me her "miracle baby" because I'm still around. I guess I'm just lucky, but I don't remember that at all. Those are the only big diseases I've had."

"Well, those are unusual. You're probably pretty lucky to be here. Have you had any surgeries in your past?"

"**No**, I sure haven't."

"I know you said you go to college. Does that mean you've gotten all your immunizations?"

"Oh, **yeah**."

"Are you allergic to anything?"

"**Grass**. I get **hay fever** in the summer when people cut their lawns. **Otherwise, nothing**."

Return to prior symptoms or subjects if clarification is needed.

Make a strong effort to respond to the patient's points. Be easy to talk to, rather than just an interviewer.

25

"Are you on any medications now?"

"Actually, I take a medicine called **minocycline** for **acne**. I forgot that. I take that every day. In the summertime, I also take a **pill** to help my **allergies**, I'm not on that right now, though."

"Are you taking anything for that arthritis?"

"**No**, I don't need to."

"When exactly was that last flare-up?"

"Oh, I haven't had one since I was about 14 years old. I was in the eighth grade. That's it."

"Ok. How about smoking or use of tobacco?"

"I **smoke** sometimes when I go out with my friends."

"Do you drink alcohol at all?"

"I've tried it, but **I don't really like it**. I've **gotten drunk a couple times,** but it doesn't make me feel very good so I don't drink."

"Ok. How about other drugs?"

"**Nope**."

"Alright. Does anyone in your family have any major diseases?"

"My mom has **lupus**. She has good times and bad, but she's doing alright. My dad is alright, too. He has **high cholesterol** and **diabetes**—the kind you have to take **insulin for**. But otherwise, they're ok."

Signpost for the Physical Exam

"Ok. I'd like to do a physical exam now, if you don't mind. Just let me **wash my hands.** First I'd like to take a look at your eyes…"

Objective

Points for Every Exam:

- Wash hands.
- Comment on vital signs, even if normal.
- Tell the patient where you are going to examine and disrobe.
- Do not repeat painful maneuvers.

Physical Exam:

Perform a focused physical, by system, from the head down.

System	Exam elements	Findings in this patient
HEENT	Test the visual fields and peripheral vision as well as extra-ocular muscle movements. Use a Snellen eye chart to determine visual acuity of the affected eye. Examine the pupil reactivity and comment on external ocular abnormities.	Eyes: PERRLA, extra-ocular muscles intact. Right scleral injection. No visible foreign body. No focal erythema or subconjunctival hemorrhage. Vision is unable to be determined in affected eye.
Retina	Use an ophthalmoscope to examine both retina. Change focus to examine anterior chamber/lens then focus on the retina.	No visible abnormalities on model patient.

Continue to gather information as you do the physical exam. Comment aloud on any real or simulated abnormalities.

Example: *"Please allow me to look underneath your eyelid. This may be somewhat uncomfortable, but tell me if you have pain. I plan to invert the upper lid…[while using end of Q-tip to roll the upper lid to the inverted position]."*

Example: *"I know this light can be bright, and this exam is uncomfortable because of that. Please bear with me, though, because it is really important that I see your eye clearly."*

End of Case

End by explaining you have several ideas of what could be wrong and could cause these symptoms. Tell the patient the first two diagnoses on your differential list and the major tests you'd now like to perform.

TABLE 2.1 Differential Diagnosis of "Red Eye"

	Conjunctiva	Iris	Pupil	Cornea	Anterior chamber	Intraocular pressure	Appearance
Acute glaucoma	Both ciliary and conjunctival vessels injected Entire eye is red	Injected	Dilated, fixed, oval	Steamy, hazy	Very shallow	Very high	
Anterior Uveitis	Redness most marked around cornea Color does not blanch on pressure	Injected	Small, fixed	Normal	Turgid	Normal	
Conjunctivitis	Conjunctival vessels injected, greatest toward fornices Blanch on pressure Mobile over sclera	Normal	Normal	Normal	Normal	Normal	
Subconjunctival haemorrhage	Bright red sclera with white rim around limbus	Normal	Normal	Normal	Normal	Normal	

Oxford Handbook of Clinical Medicine, Longmore, Wilkinson, © 2004, OUP 6th Ed.

Example: *"Ms. Eathe, there are several eye problems that might explain your symptoms. One is called 'uveitis' which is an inflammatory process of the front part of the eye. It sometimes happens in people for unknown reasons or is associated with bigger diseases, such as juvenile or children's arthritis, which may be a cause in your case. This disease has a lot of features that you describe and is one I'm considering today. The best way to evaluate for this is by looking at your eye with a special magnifier called a slit lamp. It's pretty simple and something I can do in the office. If I see something that suggests this is a possibility, I'll have to have you see an eye specialist. Another possibility is that you have what you referred to earlier as 'pink eye' or conjunctivitis. That's when the outer part of the eye gets irritated either by infection with bacteria or a virus or it is allergic. As well as these possibilities, you might also have a small piece of dirt or something we call a 'foreign body' in the outer layer that is still causing you a problem. Sometimes these 'foreign bodies' can actually cause a little cut or abrasion to the surface of the eye that can also cause this sort of reaction. I'll test for this possibility by placing a small drop of* *orange dye in your eye and looking at it with that slit lamp magnifier I talked about before. Please let me step out and arrange for these exams with my nurse so we can get started.*

Before I go, is there any other aspect of your health care we haven't already discussed? Ok then, thank you."

PATIENT NOTE

History: Include significant positives and negatives from history of present illness, past medical history, review of system(s), social history, and family history.

HPI: 19 y/o female with 1-week history of red, irritated right eye. Onset occurred after playing sports outside in the wind and has worsened over the interim. Symptoms include unilateral redness, 5/10 pain described as foreign body-like sensation progressing to a dull ache, tearing, photophobia, and blurring of vision. Pain does not radiate but is worse in bright environments. Pt admits to history of conjunctivitis of shorter duration and allergies to grass in the summer.

PMH: Meningitis, juvenile rheumatoid arthritis, acne vulgaris, seasonal allergies.

PSH: None.

Tobacco: Denies.

EtOH: Socially rarely.

Meds: Minocycline.

FamH: Mother-SLE. Father-IDDM, hypercholesterolemia.

Physical Examination: Indicate only pertinent positive and negative findings related to the patient's chief complaint.

VS stable. HEENT: Eyes: PERLA, extraocular muscles intact. No hemorrhages or focal erythema. No visible foreign body. Visual acuity unable to be determined in the affected eye.

Retina: Undilated exam: Normal retina without signs of edema, vessel abnormalities, or blurring of the optic disc. Suboptimal exam due to undilated state.

Differential Diagnosis: In order of likelihood (with 1 being the most likely), list up to 5 potential or possible diagnoses for this patient's presentation (in many cases, fewer than 5 diagnoses are likely)	Diagnostic Work-up: List immediate plans (up to 5) for further diagnostic work-up
1. Anterior uveitis	1. Slit lamp and dilated eye exam
2. Viral conjunctivitis	2. Florescence eye exam
3. Bacterial conjunctivitis	3. CBC with differential, renal function testing
4. Foreign body or corneal abrasion	4. HLA-B27 testing
5. Closed angle glaucoma	5. Tonometry

1. Opening Scenario

Jack Plaster, a 78-year-old male, has come to the office with complaints of memory loss. His wife is accompanying him.

2. Vital Signs

BP: 128/88 mmHg

Temp: 98.6° F (37.0° C)

HR: 72/minute, regular

RR: 12/minute

3. Examinee Tasks

1. Obtain a focused history.

2. Perform a relevant physical examination. (Do not perform breast, pelvic/genital, or rectal examination.)

3. Discuss your initial diagnostic impression and your work-up plan.

4. After leaving the room, complete your patient note on the given form.

Are the Vital Signs Stable?

Subjective

Knock; enter. Introduce yourself, and place the first signpost.

"Hello Mr. and Mrs. Plaster, I'm Dr. Jenson. I understand you've had some trouble with memory, Mr. Plaster. Please tell me more about it."

Mr. Plaster: "Hello, doctor. Good to see you. Yeah, I've been having more problems than usual lately. Sherry thinks I've been **getting worse**. I've had a **bad memory** now for a long time. Everybody knows that, but she says I've gotten worse."

Mrs. Plaster: "Yes, I just want to say I've noticed Bill's been **asking a lot of questions that he should know the answer to,** you know. It just seems like he doesn't know familiar places or some things anymore. For instance, he seems like he's **gotten lost** a lot lately. He sometimes does that, and that's why I'm the one that drives us everywhere. Whenever we go out to the store, or library, or whatever,

I'm just not sure he knows the way. He's driven us to the wrong place a few times, and so I just started driving. He also tells me he's **unsteady when he walks**. That's the new problem. It's like he needs to **hold onto things** as he walks around the house. I guess he's just getting older, but all these things together make me concerned."

"Bill, what do you think about what your wife just said? Do you get lost a lot and feel like you don't know where you are?"

Mr. Plaster: "**Yeah**, I do. I've lived in my home now for 26 years and left to walk to the store yesterday and **forgot my way back**. I've never had that problem before. Hell, the store's only a block away. I almost had to go into a house and ask 'Can I use your phone to call my wife to come pick me up?' It's embarrassing. It's like someone dropped me off in a strange neighborhood. It's not all the time, but sometimes it happens."

"How about asking your wife questions you might feel you once knew the answer to?"

Mr. Plaster: "Well, I've always done that. She thinks it's more, but I do that and I've always done that."

Mrs. Plaster: "He's always let me keep track of things, especially when paying the bills and things, but he asked me the other day if we banked at a bank that's on the corner of our street. We've been going to that bank for 20 years. He's always known that's where we go. So that's something. Then about a week ago, he asked what our **cat's name** was. It was late, when we were going to bed, but he's the one who named the cat. He used to know her. Since then, he's remembered, but it's just strange for him to not know these things."

"Yes, I would think it would be somewhat strange. Mr. Plaster, can you tell me about needing to hold onto things when you walk?"

Mr. Plaster: "Yeah, well, I need to **hold onto things** when I walk now. I'm retired with the post office. Twenty-eight years I was a **mail carrier**. Now it feels like I might fall if I try to walk around my house sometimes. I just feel **unsteady**."

"Do you feel dizzy?"

Mr. Plaster: "**No**, not exactly, it's more of feeling unsteady. I **don't feel dizzy,** I just feel like if I don't hold onto something I might fall."

"Have you ever fallen?"

Mr. Plaster: "There was that time a year ago when I **fell** at Christmastime. I fell on the ice. Doctor said I was lucky I didn't break anything."

"How about lately?"

Mr. Plaster: "**No**. This is only about the last few weeks I've felt like this."

"Ok. Have you started any new medicines since these symptoms began?"

Mrs. Plaster: "No he hasn't doctor."

Mr. Plaster: "Nope I haven't."

"What medications are you taking?"

Mrs. Plaster: "His regular doctor has him taking **Atenolol** and **Lisinopril** for his **high blood pressure**; he takes **lovastatin** for **high cholesterol**,

> When a patient with suspected dementia is present, try to ask questions directly of them.

tamsulosin for his **prostate**, and **glyburide** for his **diabetes**. I do all his medicines. We have a daily routine, and I make sure both of us get our medicines on time."

"Is that a change that you organize his medications, or has that always been the case?"

Mrs. Plaster: "I've **always** done that for him. I set out the whole week, and because I'm on some medicines, too, I just do them both at the same time."

"How long has he had memory problems?"

Mrs. Plaster: "It's been a while now. I'd say it's been a **couple of years** he's had it building. I mean, he hasn't had trouble finding his way around until, maybe, the last couple of **months**, but he's had problems for years."

"Has he ever forgotten your name or the name of his children?"

Mrs. Plaster: "**No**, I can't say he has. He looks at the neighbors like they're unfamiliar from time to time, but I don't know. He hasn't forgotten my name."

Mr. Plaster: "Yeah, sometimes it takes me a minute if someone comes to the door. That feeling is really uncomfortable."

"I can imagine how that would feel. Are there any other symptoms lately that you'd like to discuss? Things that may have started happening along with his memory problems and unsteadiness while walking?"

Mrs. Plaster: "No, that's it. Do you think it's something like **Alzheimer's** disease?"

"Well, I can't say what it might be at this point. Alzheimer's is a concerning disease that may have some of the same features that you're describing, but it's too early to tell that now. Alzheimer's and other diseases that cause what's called 'dementia' are often hard to diagnose. Before making that diagnosis I'd like to ask more questions and do some tests. It's possible that if we're able to find the reason for these symptoms that it may be reversible, in which case we could certainly treat it. I'd like to ask a few more questions so I can figure out what tests we should run, ok? Have you had any problems moving your arms or legs recently?"

Mr. Plaster: "Oh, **no**. I can move just fine."

"Ok. How about feeling? Do you have any numbness or unusual sensations in your body?"

Mr. Plaster: "**No**, it's like it always is. My doctor pokes me with that little filament every time I come see him to check my diabetes. I can still feel fine."

"I know you said earlier you don't feel dizzy and that you fell down that once. Do you ever lose consciousness without meaning to?"

Mr. Plaster: "**Nope**."

"Do you have any new problems seeing?"

Mr. Plaster: "**No**, I've used these same glasses for 10 years now."

"Alright. How about any chest pain?"

Mr. Plaster: "**No**, no. I'd tell a doctor right away if that happened."

> Answering direct questions honestly regarding patient's fears during the interview is important. If need be, explain the plan to evaluate for the specific disease and inform them about it.

"Any trouble breathing?"

Mr. Plaster: "**No**, never have."

"Do you ever get pain in your feet or legs? Especially when walking?"

Mr. Plaster: "**No**. I don't get pain down there. Remember, I'm a mail carrier."

"Do you ever have pain in your abdomen or trouble eating?"

Mr. Plaster: "I eat like a horse—ask my wife!"

Mrs. Plaster: "He eats just fine. **No problems**; he always has."

"Any problems going to the bathroom?"

Mr. Plaster: "**No**, I really pay attention to eating fruit every day. Keeps me regular, ya know."

"Ok. How about urinating? I know you're on a medicine for your prostate. Any problems getting to the bathroom in time?"

Mr. Plaster: "Actually, yeah. I have **dribbled on myself** a few times."

"Has that been because you didn't get to the bathroom in time or because you didn't feel like you had to go?"

Mr. Plaster: "I didn't know I had to, actually. I did that last week actually. Just sitting watching TV and felt wet. Didn't even feel like I had to go."

Mrs. Plaster: "He did, actually. It wasn't a whole lot of pee but enough to have to change. I forgot about that."

"How about starting a stream of urine? Is that difficult?"

Mr. Plaster: "**Not** now, it's not. Doctor put me on that medicine and it helps pretty well. When I first had that big prostate he put me on the medicine and it worked pretty well."

"Ok. So when you have to go to the bathroom to urinate, do you feel like you better hurry or you'll lose control?"

Mr. Plaster: "**No**, I have enough warning."

"How about any burning when you urinate?"

Mr. Plaster: "I don't have that."

"Alright. Any fever lately?"

Mr. Plaster: "**No**, not at all."

"Ok. I know about your medicines, can you tell me about what medical problems you have?"

Mr. Plaster: "Well, I've got **high blood pressure**, **high cholesterol**, a **big prostate**, and **that other thing…diabetes**. I take medicine for all of them. I had some corns on my feet, too, for years, but I got an operation and they're gone."

"Have you had any other operations?"

Mrs. Plaster: "He was **shot** when he was in the war. It **broke his leg,** and he was operated on then. Otherwise, no."

"Do you remember that Mr. Plaster?"

"Oh **sure**, I remember that. Ha, that was one hell of a time Doc. The world doesn't have wars like the Big One anymore."

"Alright. Do you now or have you ever smoked?"

Mrs. Plaster: "**No** he hasn't."

"How about drink alcohol?"

Mr. Plaster: "Used to as a younger man, but I've not been a drinker in 30 years. It's nice every now and then, but I only touch it rarely."

"Alright. Are there any other diseases in your family?"

Mr. Plaster: "**No**, the kids are healthy. I don't think they even have any worries. My son's in law school and my daughter just had her third daughter. Her name is…Sherry, what's….Sherry, what'd they name the baby?"

Mrs. Plaster: "They named her Emily, Bill. Emily."

"Is that the type of thing that's easy for you to forget?"

Mr. Plaster: "**Yeah**, sorry. It happens at the damndest times. Emily…"

"Ok. Have there been any diseases causing memory problems in your parents or other family members?"

Mr. Plaster: "I don' think so."

Mrs. Plaster: "No, I don't believe so."

Signpost for the Physical Exam

"Ok. I'd like to do a physical exam now, if you don't mind. Just let me **wash my hands**. It looks like your **vital signs are normal,** so please let me first look in your ears…"

Objective

Points for Every Exam:

- Wash hands.
- Comment on vital signs, even if normal.
- Tell the patient where you are going to examine and disrobe.
- Do not repeat painful maneuvers.

Physical Exam:

Perform a focused physical, by system, from the head down.

System	Exam elements	Findings in this patient
HEENT	Ears: check TMs visually and with insufflator bulb, Eye: Check pupillary light reflexes.	TM's are pearly grey bilaterally, normal mobility, no external ear or mastoid tenderness, Eyes were PERRLA, EOM's are intact. Rest of HEENT exam was normal.
Neuro	Assess cranial nerves and tactile sensation of the extremities including using a monofilament. Test digital proprioception. Perform sharp/dull testing. Test motor strength of the extremities and deep tendon reflexes. Ask the patient to perform dysdiadochokinesis. Perform a detailed gait assessment, including heel-walk and toe-walk. Make sure to be able to catch the patient if he falls. Assess special testes such as Romberg's sign, finger-to-nose, heel-to-shin, and Babinski's sign. Check for ankle clonus.	Tactile sensation and monofilament negative. Motor 5/5, symmetric, CN's II-XII intact. Proprioception intact, Dysdiadochokinesis normal, Gait unsteady and broad-based. Unable to complete heel- and toe-walk. DTRs, 2+ and symmetric. Romberg sign negative. Finger-to-nose and heel-to-shin, normal. Babinski's downgoing. No tremor. One beat of clonus.
Heart	Listen to 4 different auscultation areas on chest. Listen for carotid bruit's. Check peripheral pulses.	Regular rate and rhythm. No murmurs, rubs, gallups. No carotid bruit's. Pulses 2+ and symmetric.

Continue to gather information as you do the physical exam. Ask about pertinent aspects of each system as you perform the exams. Comment aloud on any real or simulated abnormalities.

Example: *"When you close your eyes, do you feel like you might fall?"*

Example: *"Do you have any pain in your ears?"*

End of Case

End by explaining you have several ideas of what could be wrong and could cause these symptoms. Tell the patient the first two diagnoses on your differential list and the major tests you'd now like to perform.

Example: *"Mr. and Mrs. Plaster, I can't tell exactly what might be going on to cause these symptoms. However, there are some tests I'd like to run to try to find out. One possibility is a disease that's called 'normal pressure hydrocephalus,' which is a fancy name for when the fluid that normally bathes the brain builds up there and is a cause of harm. This disease is thankfully reversible and may be causing what is going on here, but the best way to tell is an MRI, or brain scan, to look at the brain itself. The test itself is pretty easy in that you'll have to lie on a small table, which then moves in and out of a tunnel like machine. It takes pictures of your brain as you move in and out. Another possibility, like we talked about before, is the onset of Alzheimer's disease. This is a concerning disease that can cause some of the memory-type symptoms you have. It's a common disease, but there is really no excellent way to tell if that's the cause. For this one, I want to eliminate other possibilities before pointing to it because Alzheimer's isn't totally curable, although we do have medicines to help. Overall, I will have to take some blood today, some urine today, do a quick genital and prostate exam, and have you followed up for that brain scan at the radiology department. Please allow me to step out and arrange for those tests while I have you step into a gown.*

Is there any other aspect of your health care we haven't already discussed? Ok then, thank you."

PATIENT NOTE

History: Include significant positives and negatives from history of present illness, past medical history, review of system(s), social history, and family history.

HPI: 78 y/o male presents with his wife and caregiver, with c/o increasing forgetfulness, unfamiliarity with surroundings, and unsteady gait. Time-course has been months in the development with recent and gradual worsening. Forgetfulness is seen as inability to drive and recognize the neighborhood and forgetting proper names. +Unsteady gait, especially around the house and needs assistance. One incident of a fall 1 year ago, but question of slipping on ice. Pt denies other neurologic complaints such as vertigo, eyesight difficulties, decreased sensation, decreased motor, or focal neurologic effects.

ROS: Incontinence of urine. O/w negative urinary symptoms.

Meds: Atenolol, lisinopril, lovastatin, glyburide, tamsulosin.

PMH: Hypertension, hypercholesterolemia, type II diabetes, BPH.

PSH: Foot corn removal, gunshot wound—historic.

Smoking: Denies.

Alcohol use: Rarely.

FamH: Noncontributory.

Physical Examination: Indicate only pertinent positive and negative findings related to the patient's chief complaint.

VS Stable, normal.

Neuro: Tactile sensation and monofilament normal. CN's II–XII intact. Motor 5/5 and symmetric, Proprioception intact, dysdiadochokinesis normal, unassisted gait unsteady with broad base. Unable to complete heel- and toe-walks. DTRs 2+ and symmetric. Romberg negative. Finger-to-nose normal, Heel to shin, normal. Babinski's sign downgoing. No tremor. No pathologic clonus.

HEENT: Ears: TMs pearly gray bilaterally, no effusion, erythema. Normal movement. Eyes: PERRLA.

Heart: RRR no murmurs, rubs, gallops. Pulse's normal. No carotid bruit's.

Differential Diagnosis: In order of likelihood (with 1 being the most likely), list up to 5 potential or possible diagnoses for this patient's presentation (in many cases, fewer than 5 diagnoses are likely)	Diagnostic Work-up: List immediate plans (up to 5) for further diagnostic work-up
1. Normal pressure hydrocephalus	1. CBC with differential
2. Alzheimer's disease	2. MRI, brain
3. Delirium caused by occult infection	3. Genital and prostate exam
4. Multiple infarct dementia	4. Electrolyte panel and renal function
5. Parkinson's disease/dementia	5. Urine analysis and culture

4   Dizziness

Are the Vital Signs Stable?

Subjective

Knock; enter. Introduce yourself, and place the first signpost.

"Hello Ms. Castroski, I'm Dr. Schulz. I understand you've had some dizziness lately. Please tell me more about it."

"Hi doctor. Yeah, it's hard to describe, but I've been having this **dizziness** for the last **week**. It's sort of like a **constant** uneasy and dizzy feeling. Then I'll have these times here I'm more dizzy and it's very **hard to even move around the room**, you know? It's very strange."

Transition statement of empathy

"Alright, that sounds miserable. I know you said this started last week—was there any event you can point to or any cause that might have touched this off?"

"You know, I've been thinking of that too and can't figure anything out. It came on 7 days ago, pretty much **when I woke up**. It wasn't very intense but it was there a little bit, just a little. Then I went **swimming** with my friend, like I do with her every weekend, and it **got worse in the water**. I said to my friend 'I don't know what's happening to me. I must be seasick.' So then I went home, and it was still there."

"Interesting. Does the dizziness come with a full feeling in your ear or ear pain?"

"**No**, at first I thought I might have gotten water in my ear, but **it doesn't feel full**."

"About the dizziness itself—does it feel like you're spinning around the room or that the room is spinning around you?"

"Well, it's sort of like **the room is spinning around**. Like I need to stick my arms out to keep from falling. Like when you were a kid and you rolled down a hill, ya know?"

"Have you had any nausea or vomiting?"

"Not really. That first day, I think I felt a **little nauseous** on the drive home from the pool, though."

"Is this feeling any worse or better when you lie down?"

"Well, it's a **little better,** I think. Sometimes, I'll be in bed and I think it's totally gone, but then when I get up it comes back."

"But you said sometimes it's more intense than others?"

"**Yeah**, I get these times when it's **worse** and I feel really unsteady, but then, like I said, when I lay down, it sometimes gets better."

"Ok. Have you had any recent illness lately?"

"**No**, nothing really. I had a **cold** about 3 weeks ago, but that's been done for a while."

"Do you ever have allergies?"

"Oh, I get **hayfever** in the **summer and spring,** but that's normal for me. I take an allergy medicine. I'm on it now; it's called **loratadine**. But that's for my eyes and nose mainly. Allergies never caused this."

"Ok. That's only one possibility I'm thinking of. How about any other changes in your health?"

"**No**, I've been good. I'm on a few medicines for **blood pressure** and **diabetes,** but that's not a change."

"What medicines would those be?"

"I'm on **atenolol** for my blood pressure and **metformin** for diabetes. I've been on both for a while now."

"Because you're diabetic, have your blood sugars been normal recently?"

"**Yes**, they've been in the normal range. I check about **once a day**. Then I'm also on the loratadine but only because of my allergies."

"Do you take insulin for your diabetes as well?"

"**No**, I never have."

Even distant rhinitis symptoms may contribute to inflammation, which may lead to labrynthitis.

Acute illness often increases regular blood sugar values.

"Ok. Have you noticed any other symptoms lately, such as not being able to move one part of your body or another or perhaps numbness anywhere?"

"**No**, none of that."

"Any headaches at all?"

"Well, I do have a **headache**. That's another thing; I've had this headache for a few days, too, maybe the whole week now that I think about it. It's sort of constant."

"Where is the pain?"

"Sort of **all over** [pointing to her whole head]. Not one place or another—just all over generally."

"Is this type of headache unusual for you?"

"**Yeah**, I sometimes get a headache when I'm tired, but they go away with sleeping. This one has just hung around."

"Ok. Have you had any vision changes?"

"**No**, not at all."

"Are there any others in your family that have been sick?"

"**No**, my mom passed away 2 years ago of a heart attack, and my dad died about 10 years ago of a blood clot in his lungs. I used to be married but am now divorced. My two children are grown and healthy."

"Ok. Have you had any other major diseases in your life other than high blood pressure, allergies, and diabetes?"

"**No**, that's it."

"Have you ever had surgery at all?"

"**No**, never. Even both my deliveries were normal."

"Do you smoke or use tobacco in any way?"

"No, my parents smoked, and I can't stand the smell."

"How about alcohol? Do you drink?"

"I have a few drinks with my friends when we go out but only rarely. Maybe twice a month or so."

> A headache in the patient coupled with high blood pressure may be an indication that the blood pressure is present at times other than just in the office.

Signpost for the Physical Exam

"Ok. I'd like to do a physical exam now, if you don't mind. Just let me **wash my hands.** I'd first like to start by examining your ears…"

Objective

Points for Every Exam:

- Wash hands.
- Comment on vital signs, even if normal.
- Tell the patient where you are going to examine and disrobe.
- Do not repeat painful maneuvers.

Physical Exam:

Perform a focused physical, by system, from the head down.

System	Exam elements	Findings in this patient
HEENT	Examine the ears using an insufflator bulb. Comment aloud on the cone of light or any bulging or retraction of the tympanic membrane. Eyes: examine pupillary light reactivity with an ophthalmoscope, then proceed with a retinal exam. Make sure to focus on the optic disc and make a comment about blurring of the optic disc, or lack thereof. Examine the nose and throat briefly.	Ears: normal TMs bilaterally. No bulging or retractions. Cone of light anterior and normal. Normal mobility. Eyes: PERRLA, EOM's intact. Retina: normal bilaterally. Optic disc normal appearing. Nose: normal. Throat: normal.
Neck	Examine the anterior and posterior lymph node chains, commenting aloud on any abnormalities. Note ROM and any nuchal rigidity.	No lymphadenopathy noted. No nuchal rigidity noted.
Neurologic	Complete a cranial nerve exam, assess Babinski's sign, Romberg's sign, and finger-to-nose testing. Test tactile sense of all extremities followed by proprioception and sharp/dull sense. Assess deep tendon reflexes and motor strength. Observe gait, including heel- and toe-walks. Check for ankle clonus.	CN's II-XII intact. No focal signs of deficit. Normal sensation and motor control. Negative Romberg's, downgoing Babinski's, normal finger-to-nose and gait testing. No clonus.

Continue to gather information as you do the physical exam. Comment aloud on any real or simulated abnormalities.

Example: *"Does your neck hurt when you turn it from side to side?"*

Example: *"I'm sorry I have to use such a bright light during this exam. Does this make your headache worse or hurt your eyes at all?"*

End of Case

End by explaining you have several ideas of what could be wrong and could cause these symptoms. Tell the patient the first few diagnoses on your differential list and the major tests you'd now like to perform.

Example: *"Ms. Castroski, your symptoms and physical exam make me think of several possibilities that may be causing your dizziness. Because dizziness may be caused by an abnormality of either the tiny organs that help you sense your position in space that are located in the inner ear and also the brain itself, I'm going to recommend we get a test to look at those structures. To directly look at these, the best test is called an MRI, which is a type of imaging test that allows cross-section photographs of your brain to be taken. It's a generally well-tolerated procedure that involves lying on a flat table that then moves into and out of a long donut-shaped machine. It should be pretty easy for you and can show me both your tiny inner ear structures and the rest of your brain. The reason to get this is that you might have experienced a small stroke that can give you a feeling of dizziness. This is important to know because we may be able to prevent other ones from occurring if indeed that did happen. That's the most concerning of scenarios although not the only one. Another possibility is something called 'labyrinthitis,' which is inflammation occurring in that inner ear cavity that contains those tiny organs that provide your brain with position information. Also, I'd like to try another maneuver on you today to diagnose another possibility called 'benign*

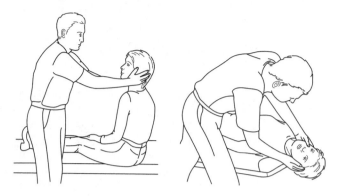

FIGURE 4.1 Dix-Hallpike maneuver.

Reprinted with permission from Manji. *Oxford Handbook of Neurology.* Oxford University Press, 2007.

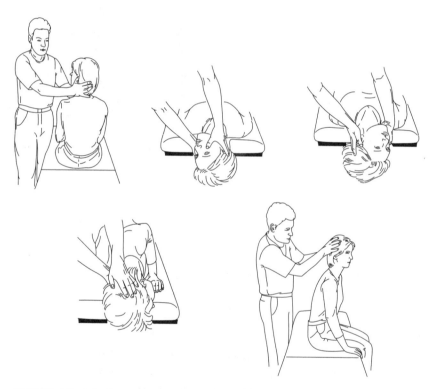

FIGURE 4.2 Epley's maneuver. Treatment of left posterior canal BPPV.

Reprinted with permission from Manji. *Oxford Handbook of Neurology.* Oxford University Press, 2007.

paroxysmal positional vertigo,' which consists of a certain abnormality of those position-sensing inner ear organs. It's something I can perform right here in the office and is a very simple change in position for you while I assess any new symptoms. Besides these tests, I'd also like to order a few routine blood tests both for screening purposes and to tell if there are other possible problems occurring in your body that might explain your symptoms. Before we get started with that maneuver, please allow me to step out and arrange these other tests with my nurse.

Before I go, is there any other aspect of your health care we haven't already discussed? Ok then, thank you."

PATIENT NOTE

History: Include significant positives and negatives from history of present illness, past medical history, review of system(s), social history, and family history.

HPI: 61 y/o female with c/o dizziness for 7 days. Onset was upon waking and has been constant baseline with episodes of worsening unrelated to identifiable cause. Pt identifies swimming activity the day of onset but states symptoms present before this activity. Last URI approximately 3 weeks prior to symptoms and is now resolved. Seasonal allergies active but symptoms treated successfully with loratadine and dizziness not indicative. Generalized, low-level headache is also present without recent worsening, although its unrelenting nature is unusual. Mild nausea present at onset but none since; patient denies other symptoms.

PMH: URI 3 wks ago. Hypertension. Seasonal allergies. Type II diabetes.

PSH: Denies.

Tobacco: Denies.

EtOH: Occasional.

Meds: Loratadine, atenolol, metformin.

Physical Examination: Indicate only pertinent positive and negative findings related to the patient's chief complaint.

VS Stable. Increased blood pressure noted.

HEENT: Ears: TMs pearly gray bilaterally. No TM retraction or bulging. Normal mobility. Cone of light anterior and normal. Eyes: PERLA, retina normal without blurred optic discs or vessel abnormalities. Nose: normal. Throat: normal.

Neck: No palpable lymphadenopathy. No nuchal rigidity.

Neuro: CN's II-XII intact. Strength 5/5 throughout, tactile sensation intact, Reflexes 2+ throughout. Proprioception normal. Sharp/dull normal. Heel- and toe-walks normal. Downgoing Babinski's sign and Romberg's sign normal. No pathologic clonus.

Differential Diagnosis: In order of likelihood (with 1 being the most likely), list up to 5 potential or possible diagnoses for this patient's presentation (in many cases, fewer than 5 diagnoses are likely)	Diagnostic Work-up: List immediate plans (up to 5) for further diagnostic work-up
1. Cerebrovascular accident (stroke)	1. MRI, brain
2. Benign paroxysmal positional vertigo	2. Dix-Hallpike maneuver
3. Labyrinthitis	3. CBC with differential
4. Diabetic neuropathy	4. Basic metabolic panel
5. Meniere's disease	5. Hemoglobin A1C

5   Headache

1. Opening Scenario

Ami Carson, a 32-year-old female, presents to the physician's office for headache.

2. Vital Signs

BP: 140/92 mmHg

Temp: 98.6° F (37.0° C)

HR: 64/minute, regular

RR: 12/minute

3. Examinee Tasks

1. Obtain a focused history.

2. Perform a relevant physical examination. (Do not perform breast, pelvic/genital, or rectal examination.)

3. Discuss your initial diagnostic impression and your work-up plan.

4. After leaving the room, complete your patient note on the given form.

Are the Vital Signs Stable?

Subjective

Knock; enter. Introduce yourself, and place the first signpost.

"Hi Ms. Carson, I'm Dr. Branson. I understand you've come in today for head-aches you've been having. Please tell me more about them."

"Hi, Dr. Branson. Yeah, I'm here because of my **horrible headaches**. I call them migraines, but I don't know. I only have them now and then, but when I have them they hurt really, really bad. I had **one start yesterday,** and it **still hurts**. It started for no real good reason, like usual, and it seems like it **hurts more at night**. I've taken **Tylenol** and **ibuprofen,** but **they don't help**. It just seems like I'm wasting my time taking those medicines. I finally need someone to do something for it all."

Transition statement of empathy

"That must be hard to take. Being in physical pain can make a lot of things in life seem so much harder. Please allow me to ask some questions and try to

42

get more of the story. I'll try to figure out what's going on and hopefully will be able to tackle this with a medicine. Severe headaches can exist because of several reasons. Can I ask how long you've been having these headaches altogether?"

"I've had them for probably **3 years**, since **my youngest was born**. I had headaches before that, but they stopped during my pregnancy. These seem **different**, though; they're longer and much more intense when they come on."

"How long do they last when they come on?"

"It **depends**. They could be, maybe, **half a day** at the shortest to a **couple of days**."

"How often would you say you get them?"

"Um, maybe **once a week**. I may go for a month without one, though. If they're really bad, I might get two in a week. That's the thing—I've been getting more and more of them lately. Last week I had one that lasted for 3 days. And the week before, I had two long ones. This week, it's Tuesday, and I've had this headache since yesterday."

"Have you found anything that tends to trigger them, such as bright lights or certain smells?"

"**No**. Once when I was coming home from a holiday with my kids, I was driving for something like 8 hours, and I thought the one that I got that night was from all the lights on the highway. Normally, I can't say there's any one trigger, though."

"Do these ever come on in relation to any part of your menstrual cycle?"

"**Maybe**. I seem to get more just **before my period**. I've wondered that, too, and I think I get more then. But I **also get headaches at other times**. I can't say it's a strong correlation."

"Are these headaches preceded by any type of vision change or warning at all?"

"**No**. You mean like a bright light?"

"Well, or anything such as seeing lights that aren't there to smelling a particular scent that might not be there. This would be called an 'aura,' which may happen before the onset of pain in certain types of headaches."

"Um . . . **no**. I haven't gotten any of that."

"Ok. You said the medicine Tylenol or ibuprofen hasn't helped in the past. Does anything?"

"I just try to lie down and go to **sleep**. When I sleep it just passes the time."

"Does laying your head down change the pain at all?"

"**Not really**."

"Ok. Let me ask a little about the location of the pain. Where does it hurt in your head?"

"It hurts usually on the **right side**. I mean, right **behind my eye** mostly, but it **goes to the back**, too. It's just a throbbing that won't go away. It feels kind of **sharp up front** near my eye, then it feels like a **dull pain in the back**. Sometimes it's the whole head, if it's really bad."

> Explanation of the reason behind the question often leads to a greater understanding and ability of the patient to answer.

Intolerability to lights or sounds isn't necessarily indicative to one type of headache or another. However, triggers might give a clue to vascular headaches.

Even if you think you know the diagnosis during the interview, completely explore other possibilities.

"When the pain's there, does anything make it worse?"

"**Lights or loud noises**, definitely. I have my husband turn the TV way down if I have a headache. I can't stand noises or lights."

"When a headache comes on, how long would you say it takes to reach its peak intensity?"

"A couple of hours, I'd say, then it stays there for as long as it lasts."

"On a scale of 0 to 10, 10 being the worst pain imaginable, where would you rate the pain at its peak?"

"I'd say 8 or so out of 10."

"Do you ever have a fever with this pain?"

"I **don't think so**. I haven't taken my temperature."

"Ok. How about any other symptoms like body aches or runny nose?"

"Well, **no**. I have **allergies,** and so I have a **runny nose a lot**. I don't have body aches really."

"Do you take medicine for those allergies?"

"I take **loratadine** a lot. I don't take it all the time, but if I'm having problems, I might take it for a week or so."

"Do you ever get sinus infections?"

"**Yeah**, I used to. I haven't had one in a long time, though. I had **surgery on my sinuses** about 5 years ago, when I was in college, and it helped. I still have **allergies**, though."

"Are you having those symptoms right now?"

"**Yeah**, a little. I haven't gotten my medicine refilled in about a month, though, so I haven't taken it. My nose is kind of runny now."

"Do you ever get facial pain? Especially around the sides of the nose?"

"**No**, not really."

"When you have these headaches, do you have watering of one or both eyes?"

"**No**, not really."

"How about nausea or vomiting when you have a headache?"

"When I have a bad one, **yeah**, I feel like I could throw up. That one time when I just came home from that holiday, I threw up twice."

"I know about the loratadine, Tylenol, and ibuprofen. Do you take any other medicines?"

"I'm also on **birth control pills**. I take those once a day."

"What is the name of those?"

"They're called Ortho-cyclen. I've been on it for years."

"Alright. Do you smoke or use tobacco?"

"**No**, I used to, but I quit about a year ago. I only smoked for about 3 years."

"How about drink alcohol?"

"I still drink **every now and then**. It's not like I can go out all the time with three kids, though."

"Do you drink caffeine?"

"Yeah, I gotta have my **morning coffee**. I guess I drink a **half-a-pot in the morning**. I'm also attached to my **diet soda**. I have about **three or four** of those throughout the day. I know it's a lot, but it helps when you have three kids."

"Alright. Have you ever tried to cut down?"

"**Yeah**, and then I'm tired. I slow down when I don't have my caffeine."

"How long have you been drinking that much, would you say?"

"Oh, I've done that since my **last pregnancy**. It's been 3 years. I only had a few cups when I was pregnant."

"Ok. I understand you've had three kids, allergies, and a sinus surgery. Have you seen the doctor for other health issues in the past?"

"**No**, not really. I was treated for **acne** around my face when I was in college, but that went away. Nothing else."

"Has anyone in your family had any health issues, especially related to headaches?"

"My mom **died** when I was 14 years old. She had **breast cancer** that spread around to her other organs. My dad always said she had **migraine headaches**, though. My dad's pretty healthy, though. He works in a gym. All my kids are healthy."

> Caffeine can contribute to headache syndromes by both a use-related correlation as well as a withdrawal syndrome.

Signpost for the Physical Exam

"Ok. I'd like to do a physical exam now, if you don't mind. Just let me **wash my hands.** I'd first like to start by examining your eyes…"

Objective

Points for Every Exam:

- Wash hands.
- Comment on vital signs, even if normal.
- Tell the patient where you are going to examine and disrobe.
- Do not repeat painful maneuvers.

Physical Exam:

Perform a focused physical, by system, from the head down.

System	Exam elements	Findings in this patient
HEENT	Palpate the head, neck, and shoulders, making note of tenderness, particularly along the temporal arteries. Eyes: Examine reactivity with an ophthalmoscope then proceed with a retinal exam. Make sure to focus on the optic disc and make a comment about blurring or lack thereof.	Head: normal, atraumatic, Ears: normal. Eyes: PERRLA, Retina: normal bilaterally; no papilledema. Marked photophobia on direct retinal exam to the point of refusing the contralateral eye exam.
Neck	Examine the anterior and posterior cervical lymph node chains, commenting aloud on any abnormalities. Listen to the carotid areas for bruit's. Complete range of motion for the neck.	No lymphadenopathy, no carotid bruit's. Normal ROM. No meningeal signs.
Neurologic	Complete a cranial nerve exam, Babinski's sign, Romberg's sign, and finger-to-nose testing. Assess tactile sense of the extremities and proprioception followed by sharp/dull testing. Test the deep tendon reflexes and motor strength. Observe gait, including heel- and toe-walk.	CN's II-XII intact, normal Babinski's and Romberg's sign. Normal finger-to-nose, proprioception, gait, sensation testing, and motor strength.

Continue to gather information as you do the physical exam. Comment aloud on any real or simulated abnormalities.

Example: *"Does your neck hurt when you turn it from side to side?"*

Example: *"I'm sorry I have to use such a bright light during this exam. Does this make your headache worse or just hurt your eyes?"*

End of Case

End by explaining you have several ideas of what could be wrong and could cause these symptoms. Tell the patient the first two diagnoses on your differential list and the major tests you'd now like to perform.

Example: *"Ms. Grotts, judging from your history and the physical exam I just did, there could be several reasons you're getting these headaches. First, they may be caused by the excess caffeine you seem to be taking in every day. Caffeine, just by how it works, tends to cause blood vessels to dilate or get larger. A well-known cause of headaches is sometimes when your body doesn't get this help in dilating the vessels in your brain and they constrict, which, in turn, causes the pain. That's called a caffeine withdrawal or caffeine-related headache, and because your caffeine intake is so high, I think that's a real possibility. Another cause could be that these are migraine headaches. There are several types of migraines that really fit into a broad class of headache called 'vascular type.' That simply means the pain is caused by the nerves around the blood vessels in your head, again because of uncontrolled constriction. The types of migraine vary but may have certain similarities so that they can be treated somewhat the same. Because this is the first time you've been evaluated for these severe headaches, I'd like to get some more tests to also eliminate rare causes such as sinus infection or, very rarely, a mass in your head. This will be some blood work, and I'll also arrange a CT scan of your head. A CT scan, or "cat scan", refers to a special type of X-ray that is taken of your head and shows your brain and skull in cross-section. The test itself involves laying on a thin table, which then moves you in and out of a donut-shaped machine that takes the X-rays. I'd like to step out and arrange these tests with my nurse.*

Is there any other aspect of your health care we haven't already discussed? Ok then, thank you."

PATIENT NOTE

History: Include significant positives and negatives from history of present illness, past medical history, review of system(s), social history, and family history.

HPI: 32 y/o female c/o unilateral, throbbing headaches x 3 years. Headaches occur on average every week, although they've recently been noted to increase frequency. Pain is described as sharp behind one eye that becomes dull toward the back of the head, although global symptoms rarely occur. When pain is worst, 8/10, it's accompanied by nausea/vomiting and bilateral pain. Some relation to beginning of menses, but this timing is not consistent. Pt denies facial pain, fever, vision changes, aura. Caffeine intake—excessive with several cups coffee in A.M. and 3–4 diet sodas during the day.

PMH: Allergic rhinitis, deliveries x 3, acne.

PSH: Sinus surgery.

Tobacco: Denies.

EtOH: Occasional.

Drugs: Denies.

Meds: Loratidine, OCPs, occasional Tylenol, ibuprofen.

FamH: Mother—deceased, breast cancer, migraines; father—no problems.

Physical Examination: Indicate only pertinent positive and negative findings related to the patient's chief complaint.

VS stable. Elevated blood pressure noted.

HEENT: Head NC/AT. No muscular abnormalities in head, neck, or shoulders. Ears: TMs pearly gray bilaterally. Eyes: +photophobia, PERRLA, retina normal without blurred optic discs (limited due to photophobia).

Neck: Normal ROM. No palpable lymphadenopathy. No nuchal rigidity.

Neuro: CN's II-XII intact. Strength 5/5 throughout, tactile sensation intact, Reflexes 2+ bilaterally. Proprioception normal. Sharp/dull normal. Heel- and toe-walks normal. Babinski's/Romberg's signs normal.

Differential Diagnosis: In order of likelihood (with 1 being the most likely), list up to 5 potential or possible diagnoses for this patient's presentation (in many cases, fewer than 5 diagnoses are likely)	Diagnostic Work-up: List immediate plans (up to 5) for further diagnostic work-up
1. Caffeine-related headaches	1. CT scan, head
2. Migraine, common type	2. CT scan, sinuses
3. Migraine, menstrual-related	3. CBC with differential
4. Sinusitis	4. Basic metabolic panel
5. Tension type headache	5.

6   Sleep Difficulties

1. Opening Scenario

Pej Lei, a 33-year-old male, has come to the outpatient clinic for sleep problems.

2. Vital Signs

BP: 122/78 mmHg

Temp: 98.3° F (36.8° C)

HR: 60/minute, regular

RR: 12/minute

3. Examinee Tasks

1. Obtain a focused history.

2. Perform a relevant physical examination. (Do not perform breast, pelvic/genital, or rectal examination.)

3. Discuss your initial diagnostic impression and your work-up plan.

4. After leaving the room, complete your patient note on the given form.

Are the Vital Signs Stable?

Subjective

Knock; enter. Introduce yourself, and place the first signpost.

"Hello Mr. Lei, I'm Dr. Henney. I understand you've had some difficulty sleeping lately. Please tell me what seems to be the problem."

Transition Statement of Empathy

"Hi doctor. Yeah, I'm just having a **hard time** with **sleeping** at **night**. I go to bed and feel like I can't sleep all night, then get up in the morning tired."

"That must be frustrating. Do you feel like you're having trouble getting to sleep or staying asleep?"

"I'd say **both**, really. Maybe more trouble **getting to sleep**. I just **lie** there."

"How long would you estimate it takes you to fall asleep, if you do at all?"

"May be a **couple hours**. Every night."

"Are you sleepy in the morning when you wake up? That is, if you wanted to, could you sleep in?"

"Well…**maybe**. I've never been able to. I have to get the **kids** to school. I have two daughters and a son. I never sleep in."

"Ok. Let me ask some questions about what I call 'sleep hygiene.' It's basically what your sleep habits are and how regularly you stick to them. About what time do you go to bed at night?"

"About **11 P.M.**, I suppose. Maybe later, but that's about usual."

"Do you watch TV at all or read in bed?"

"I **watch TV** for a little while. I can't sleep without relaxing some."

"How long is the TV usually on for?"

"I set the timer, I set it for a **half an hour** when I get into bed."

"Ok. And when do you get up in the morning?"

"About **5:30 A.M**. I have to get ready, cook the kids' breakfast. I have three kids, and get ready for work myself, then I've got to have time to drive us all to where we go. Morning's my busiest time of day. But, ya know, I've always been like that. I've always been a morning person."

"Ok, that's about 6 hours set aside for sleep. Do you ever take naps during the day?"

"I wish I could. I'm an **air traffic control supervisor,** so I don't have any downtime during the day at all. When I come home from work, sometimes I watch TV with the kids and end up falling asleep, but it's only for a few minutes. My oldest, Lacy, makes dinner for us a lot."

"Well, it's nice to have that help from the kids. Do you drink coffee, tea, soda, or any other source of caffeine?"

"Yeah. I have about **two cups in the morning**. I drink **coffee**. It's not the espresso or anything—just the regular drip coffee."

"Has that changed recently?"

"**No**. It's never been more than that, I don't drink those other things."

"Ok. Let me ask some other social-type questions if you don't mind. You said before that you have to get the kids up and cook them breakfast and drive them to school. Do you have a partner to help with that?"

"**No**. We've had some problems in our family. My **wife left** us about **9 months ago**. We were fighting a lot and were talking about getting a **divorce**. Then one day I came home from work and she left a letter saying she was moving back with her mother. She even left the kids at school for me to pick up. I called her mom's house, of course, and her **mother hadn't heard from her**. She called about a month later and said she was leaving because she couldn't take the tension and that I had to take care of the kids. [tearing up] It was very hard on all of us. Lord knows it was the hardest thing I've ever had to do. I mean, how can you just leave your family? It's insane!"

"That's very hard to take for anyone. How are you doing with it?"

> Elements of Poor "Sleep Hygiene"
> Watching TV in bed
> Working in bed (such as on a laptop)
> Drinking excessive caffeine during the day
> Eating close to going to sleep
> Napping during the day
> Not allowing adequate time for sleep

> Look for a disease, not just the symptoms when seeing a patient with an otherwise unexplained complaint.

"I **do what I have to**. I'm sorry…[sniffling] I just do what I have to do. It's just the way it is. We're alright; we'll be alright. I just can't imagine what she did this for…anyway…"

"That's a really tough position to be in. I'm sorry that happened to you. It must be very difficult."

"Yeah. Well…anyway, so I've had **trouble sleeping pretty much since she left.**"

"I can imagine. I think it's very reasonable to have some problems after having your partner leave and you having to take on such a responsibility."

"Yeah, we've been getting along. I'm doing what I can right now. You know, I have to work and also keep the kids in school and stuff. I love my kids, so, I'm ok with doing it. It's just hard to do it all at once and alone."

"I'll bet. I don't expect that to be easy at all. Have you seen a counselor or Chaplain?"

"I've been talking to my **priest** at **church**. And we're **working on** a lot of this stuff. The kids are in church activities so their instructors are also talking to them. That's where they are now."

"That's good. Sometimes this type of thing can affect more than one aspect of your life. Are you having any other problems, such as eating?"

"**Yeah**, I've been eating less lately, too. I'm not hungry much."

"Some people also get the feeling that they don't look forward to things they used to when something like this happens to them. Do you ever get that feeling? That is, is it hard to look forward to things for you?"

"**Yeah**, I'm feeling a lot like that. It's been like that for about the **last month**. I used to like coming home to my family at night, you know, after the work day. Now I don't as much."

"How about concentration? Do you feel like you're still thinking clearly?"

"**Yeah**, that's alright, when I'm not distracted by something else."

"How about your level of energy every day? I know you feel like you don't sleep enough so that might also affect it."

"**Yeah**, I'm **always tired**. I have a real problem with energy."

"Ok. How about thoughts of hurting yourself? Have you ever thought about suicide or that it might be better if you weren't here?"

"**No**, I couldn't do that to my kids. We're having a rough time right now but I couldn't ever do that to them. To have two parents run out on them…that just isn't right."

"Ok. How about hurting anyone else?"

"**No**, I don't want to do that."

"Do you have anyone, such as a relative or friend, that you can talk to about what's going on?"

"Yeah, **my parents** come down to our house every other weekend or so. I talk to them and they help with the kids. My **wife's mom** also comes sometimes when she can. She feels just horrible about the whole thing. My neighbors are good, too, and they pick the kids up from school and give

> When a patient makes a confession or admits a major emotional problem, it's important to encourage dialogue and let the patient talk about his/her problems. This strengthens your relationship and allows for more accurate mental health referrals.

them dinner when I have to work late. It's no substitute for a mother, but at least everyone's helping."

"That social support network can be very helpful when people go through hard times. I'd like to ask about other aspects of your health, too. Do you drink alcohol at all?"

"**No**, I never touch it."

"How about smoke or use tobacco?"

"**No**, I don't do that either."

"Are there any other drugs you take?"

"**No**, I wouldn't do that."

"Ok. Are you on any medications?"

"I take **rizatriptan** for **migraine headaches** now and then."

"How often do you take that?"

"About **once a month** if I have a migraine. Not that often. I take **Tylenol** usually, too, if I get one."

"Ok. Are you allergic to anything?"

"**No**."

"Have you had any other health problem in the past?"

"**No**, I've never had much of a problem. I had a **root canal** last month. I also had seen my doctor a couple months ago about this thing on my leg. See the scar? [Pointing to right lower leg.] He did a biopsy and it was fine."

"Was that a skin lesion?"

"Yeah, just a small **mole** on my leg."

"Ok. Have you ever stayed the night in the hospital?"

"**Nope**, never."

"How about any diseases in your family? Does anyone in the family have health concerns?"

"**Not** really. My parents are both in publishing in California. They don't really have any health problems."

> Even if you think you have a reasonable list of differential diagnoses, don't forget other elements of the interview, i.e. past medical history or medications.

Signpost for the Physical Exam

"Ok. I'd like to do a physical exam now if you don't mind. Just let me **wash my hands**. It looks like your **vital signs are normal,** so please let me first look in your ears…"

Objective

Points for Every Exam:

- Wash hands.
- Comment on vital signs, even if normal.

- Tell the patient where you are going to examine and disrobe.
- Do not repeat painful maneuvers.

Physical Exam:

Perform a focused physical, by system, from the head down.

System	Exam elements	Findings in this patient
Thyroid	Observe the thyroid gland and ask the patient to swallow before feeling them. Then, feel for the thyroid gland with both hands while standing behind the patient. Palpate the gland as the patient swallows again.	Normal, no enlargement.

Continue to gather information as you do the physical exam. Ask about pertinent aspects of each system as you perform the exams. Comment aloud on any real or simulated abnormalities.

Example: *"When you close your eyes, do you feel like you will fall?"*

Example: *"Do you have any pain in your ears?"*

End of Case

End by explaining you have several ideas of what could be wrong and could cause these symptoms. Tell the patient the first two diagnoses on your differential list and the major tests you'd now like to perform.

Example: *"Mr. Lei, based on talking with you and doing your physical exam, there are a few things that might be causing these sleep problems. The first is a mood disorder, such as depression. You have certainly had a big stressor in your life recently and now have had to take on an enormous change. That would reasonably be expected to take a big toll on anyone. Depression is something that can affect many areas of your life, and sleep and appetite are two of them. It can certainly prevent a solid sleep schedule and, thus, cause daytime drowsiness. There are a few other possibilities for your symptoms, which include variants of depression—that is, psychological disorders related to but different than depression—or there could be something biologically wrong. A biological problem could be something like a low thyroid gland. For that, I'd like to get some blood work on you today to check. I think overall we need to ultimately get you to a mental health professional so you can be better diagnosed and treated for this problem. They can also tell more accurately what disorder you have and support you through these tough times. During this whole process, though, it's important you feel supported and know that there will always be a place for you in this clinic if you feel like you're in crisis. If you ever have thoughts of hurting yourself or someone else, know that you can always come here and we can talk about it. Before you go, I'd like to give you a list of local resources that can help if you ever feel like you're being overwhelmed. Let me step out and get those for you. I'll also arrange for my nurse to come in and draw that blood that we talked about.*

Is there any other aspect of your health care we haven't already discussed? Ok then, thank you."

PATIENT NOTE

History: Include significant positives and negatives from history of present illness, past medical history, review of system(s), social history, and family history.

HPI: 33 y/o male c/o sleep disturbance since major life event of wife leaving the family approx 9 months ago. Pt reports difficulty falling asleep and staying asleep. Concurrent symptoms include decreased appetite, decreased energy, anhydonia, and depressed mood. He reports being overwhelmed by suddenly being sole provider for three kids and having to work full-time as well as deal with the loss of his wife. He denies SI/HI. Social support consists of church personnel, his own biologic parents, his wife's mother, and neighbors. Support is, however, intermittent and unreliable. He is willing to accept help.

Meds: rizatriptan—prn. Tylenol—prn.

PMH: Migraine headaches. Suspicious skin lesion-confirmed benign by biopsy.

PSH: Dental root canal—historic; skin biopsy—historic.

Smoking: Denies.

Alcohol use: Denies.

FamH: Noncontributory.

Physical Examination: Indicate only pertinent positive and negative findings related to the patient's chief complaint.

VS Stable, normal.

General: Appears normal weight and appears stated age.

Psychiatric: Nondisheveled, Asian male appearing approximately stated age. Thought processes ordered and logical. Affect is euthymic and mood-appropriate but depressed. No tangential or magical thinking. No delusions. Denies suicidal or homicidal ideation.

Thyroid: No enlargement, no abnormalities.

Differential Diagnosis: In order of likelihood (with 1 being the most likely), list up to 5 potential or possible diagnoses for this patient's presentation (in many cases, fewer than 5 diagnoses are likely)	Diagnostic Work-up: List immediate plans (up to 5) for further diagnostic work-up
1. Major depressive episode/disorder	1. TSH, free T4
2. Dysthymia	2. CBC
3. Adjustment disorder	3. Basic Metabolic Panel
4. Bereavement	4. ECG
5. Hypothyroid	5.

1. Opening Scenario

Jon McIntyre, a 27-year-old male, presents to the emergency department for evaluation of headache and fever.

2. Vital Signs

BP:	154/90 mmHg
Temp:	100.6° F (38.1° C)
HR:	94/minute, regular
RR:	16/minute

3. Examinee Tasks

1. Obtain a focused history.

2. Perform a relevant physical examination. (Do not perform breast, pelvic/genital, or rectal examination.)

3. Discuss your initial diagnostic impression and your work-up plan.

4. After leaving the room, complete your patient note on the given form.

Are the Vital Signs Stable?

Subjective

Knock; enter. Introduce yourself, and place the first signpost.

"Hi Mr. McIntyre, I'm Dr. Dobson. I understand you've been having a fever and headache lately? Can you tell me about these?"

[speaking softly] "Yeah, doc. I'm really not doing too well. I've had this **headache** for about **3 days**. It's killing me. It's weird because I really only rarely get a headache. Anyway, so yesterday I started feeling like I had a **fever**, too. You know, **hot and then cold**, then hot. My **body aches**."

"I'm sorry to hear that you're feeling like this. Would it help if I dimmed the lights?"

"It might help a little. Thanks."

Complete simple gestures for patient comfort if possible.

[Dim the lights if possible] *"Tell me about this headache. Did it come on gradually 3 days ago or all of a sudden?"*

"It was pretty **gradual**. I work in the printing industry and I'm around these big, noisy presses all day. When I get tired they can give me a headache, you know, from the noise? And so sometimes I take a **Tylenol**. It usually helps, though, and the headache goes away. Not this time. So it stayed with me and **kept building**. Now I can hardly stand it. It's the **worst headache of my life**."

"Is the headache all over your head or on one side or another?"

"It's **all over**. Started, like, in the back of my head. It hurts **all over** though.

"I know the light is hurting your eyes, but how about loud noises?"

"**Yeah**, that's why I've missed work. Those presses really make it worse."

"Have you felt nauseated as well?"

"Yeah, I **threw up** dinner **last night**. I didn't feel like eating much, but I threw up what I did eat. I've felt **nauseated** since then, so I haven't eaten anything."

"Have you had any other problems with your abdomen such as pain or diarrhea?"

"**No**, I think it's the headache. Not the stomach."

"How about any stiffness in your neck? Does it hurt to move your head?"

[turning head from side to side] "**Yeah**, that's another thing. It is a bit stiff. Right in the **back of my neck**. Maybe it's the headache."

"Do you have any other symptoms with this headache, such as dizziness?"

"**No**, I don't want to stand up, but I'm not particularly dizzy."

"Any confusion at all? A feeling like you aren't quite sure what's going on?"

"**No**, I know I'm here talking to the doctor. I'm fine as far as that."

"Have you felt like the sensation in your arms, legs, or anywhere has decreased?"

"Uh, **no**."

"Any difficulty moving one side of your body, such as you arms or legs?"

"**No**."

"How about recent cough or chest congestion?"

"Well, I had a **cold about 2 weeks ago**. It was nothing though. Took me about a week to get over it. I was **coughing** for a while, but that went away. Nothing else."

"Did you cough anything up with the cold?"

"I was at the time, but it was only during the cold. It was like a normal cold for me."

"Have you had anything else, like a skin rash, that you've noticed?"

"**No**, nothing like that."

"Ok. Tell me about the fever. I understand you've had hot and cold spells, but when did this start?"

"the worst headache of my life" are buzz words for subarachnoid hemmorhage

Key elements in the history for meningeal complaints:
 Fever presence
 Recent source of infection (i.e., sinusitis)
 Neck ROM pain
 Neurologic impairment

"That started **last afternoon**, maybe. I just started to get achy and felt warm. I was in bed, 'cause I didn't go to work. So I woke up before dinner and had **sweat out my sheets**. Then last night, I had these times when I also **felt really cold**. Horrible night it was."

"It's very hard to go through a miserable night like that. Did you take your temperature at home?"

"**No**, I just felt hot. I think your nurse said I'm running a fever."

"Yes, it looks like it from your vital signs. Have you been around anyone with symptoms like this or a fever?"

"**No**, my brother and I live together. He goes to college but he's fine."

"Have you ever had a similar illness?"

"**Not** like this exactly. 'Course, I've had a fever and headache but never together like this."

"What other things have you seen the doctor for in your life? Especially anything you've stayed overnight in the hospital for?"

"Nothing really. I saw my doctor a few months ago for **hitting my hand** on a printing press. But that's only because my boss made me. It was no big deal. Nothing broken. Other than that, I'm pretty healthy."

"Have you had any surgeries in your life?"

"I had my appendix out about 6 years ago. Actually, I spent the night for that. Otherwise no."

"Do you take medications?"

"**No**, except the **occasional Tylenol**."

"How about any dietary supplements?"

"I take **protein** powder in the morning. It's **whey protein**. I try to keep healthy and work out a lot, too."

"Are you allergic to anything?"

"**Not** that I know of."

"Ok. Do you smoke?"

"**No**, it's not good for my workouts."

"How about drink alcohol?"

"**Yeah**, I drink on the weekends. But not to get drunk or anything. I did that in college, but now I have a beer or two occasionally."

"How many beers per week would you say?"

"About **three or four**. Maybe one or two on Friday and Saturday nights. I don't drink every weekend, though. Sometimes I'm working."

"Have you ever done any other types of drugs?"

"I smoked pot in high school. Nothing else."

"Alright. Are there any major diseases in your family?"

"**No**, I don't think so. My dad was healthy until he **died in a car crash** when he was 60 years old. A trucker hit him. My **mom's fine** and lives at home alone. My brother, Jim, lives with me, and we have a sister across town. Everyone's healthy though."

Watch for patients being reminded of prior events with subsequent questions. Alteration of the history is common.

Consider asking the CAGE questions for all those who admit to alcohol use. However, they are meant for those who admit to moderate alcohol consumption and are clinically at risk for alcohol addiction.

Signpost for the Physical Exam

"Ok. I'd like to do a physical exam now, if you don't mind. Just let me **wash my hands**. I'd first like to start by examining your eyes…"

Objective

Points for Every Exam:

- Wash hands.
- Comment on vital signs, even if normal.
- Tell the patient where you are going to examine and disrobe.
- Do not repeat painful maneuvers.

Physical Exam:

Perform a focused physical, by system, from the head down.

System	Exam elements	Findings in this patient
HEENT	Palpate the head, making note of tenderness, especially in the posterior and nuchal regions. Examine the ears with an insufflator bulb. Eyes: Examine reactivity with ophthalmoscope, then proceed with a retinal exam. Make sure to focus on the optic disc and make a comment about blurring, even if none is seen. Examine the nose and throat briefly.	Head: normal, atraumatic, Ears: pearly gray TMs bilaterally. Eyes: PERRLA, Retina: normal bilaterally. Nose: normal. Throat: normal.
Neck	Examine the anterior and posterior cervical lymph node chains, commenting aloud on abnormalities. Perform Kernigs/Brudzinski's tests. Complete range of motion for the neck.	Positive Kernig's sign. Some pain on range of motion, especially forward flexion. Brudizinski's sign indeterminate.
Lungs	Auscultate the posterior lung fields. Make sure to listen to 6 points within each lung field.	Clear to auscultation bilaterally
Neurologic	Complete the cranial nerve exam, Babinski's/Romberg's signs, and finger-to-nose testing. Assess tactile sense of extremities as well as proprioception. Test deep tendon reflexes and sharp/dull testing. Assess motor strength. Observe gait including heel- and toe-walks.	Normal exam. No focal deficits. CNs II-XII intact. Strength 5/5 throughout, DTR's 2+ throughout. Normal Babinski's and Romberg's signs. Normal finger-to-nose, tactile sense, and proprioception. Normal gait.
Skin	Ask the patient to disrobe his torso, then the lower extremities while you quickly examine for a petichial rash.	Normal

Continue to gather information as you do the physical exam. Comment aloud on any real or simulated abnormalities.

Example: *"Does your neck hurt when you turn your head from side to side?"*

Example: [During the fundoscopic exam] *"I'm sorry I have to use such a bright light during this exam. Does this make your headache worse or just hurt your eyes?"*

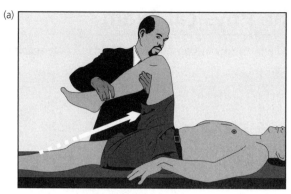

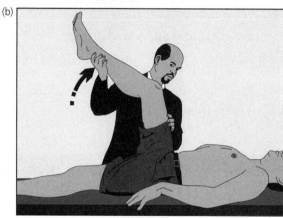

FIGURE 7.1 Eliciting Kernig's sign.

End of Case

End by explaining you have several ideas of what could be wrong and could cause these symptoms. Tell the patient the first two diagnoses on your differential list and the major tests you'd now like to perform.

Example: *"Mr. McIntyre, your symptoms are concerning me for a particular infection you may have involving the sac and fluid that surrounds the spinal cord and brain called meningitis. It's potentially a bad infection and one I think we really need to test for. The aspect of this infection that makes it particularly dangerous is that it is so close and involves the brain and spinal cord, which are very important tissues in your body. Your symptoms also could involve another type of brain abnormality that could involve bleeding of the actual brain itself, although I think this is less likely. These are the two most serious and urgent conditions I'd like to test for, and to do this I'd like to get a CT scan and then some fluid from around you spinal cord. The CT scan can show me if there is bleeding or other abnormalities of the brain, and the spinal fluid can be analyzed for signs showing infection. To obtain the spinal fluid, I'll need to do a procedure on you which involves placing a needle in the lower part of your back. It may be somewhat uncomfortable, but it really is necessary to find out if there's infection there. I'll want to get that CT scan first, however. Also, I want to obtain some blood from your vein for further testing. Please allow me to step out and arrange these tests.*

Is there any other aspect of your health care we haven't already discussed? Ok then, thank you."

PATIENT NOTE

History: Include significant positives and negatives from history of present illness, past medical history, review of system(s), social history, and family history.

HPI: 27 y/o male c/o global type headache x 3 days and fever x 24 hours. He states headache is "worst of my life" although it has progressed gradually. +neck stiffness felt mainly in posterior head and posterior/superior neck. Fever accompanied by chills and nightsweats. +Nausea and reports vomiting last meal 12 hrs ago. Moderate photophobia/phonophobia. No focal neurologic deficits. Denies rash. Most recent illness 2 wks ago described as a cold with some productive cough. No mental status changes, including dizziness or confusion.

PMH: URI 2 wks ago. Trauma to hand.

PSH: Appendectomy 6 yrs ago.

Tobacco: Denies.

EtOH: Occasional.

Drugs: Historic use marijuana.

Meds: Occasional Tylenol.

FamH: Father—deceased from trauma; mother—normal; siblings—normal.

Physical Examination: Indicate only pertinent positive and negative findings related to the patient's chief complaint.

VS Stable. Fever, elevated BP, elevated pulse noted.

HEENT: Head NC/AT, Ears: TMs normal. Eyes: PERLA, retina normal without blurred optic discs. Nose: normal. Throat: normal.

Neck: Positive nuchal rigidity. Positive Kernig's sign. Indeterminate Brudzinski's. No palpable lymphadenopathy.

Lungs: Clear to auscultation bilaterally. No wheezes/rubs/rhonchi.

Neuro: CNs II-XII intact. Strength 5/5 throughout, tactile sensation intact, Reflexes 2+ bilaterally. Proprioception normal. Sharp/dull normal. Heel- and toe-walks normal. Babinski's/Romberg's normal.

Skin: No rashes or skin lesions noted.

Differential Diagnosis: In order of likelihood (with 1 being the most likely), list up to 5 potential or possible diagnoses for this patient's presentation (in many cases, fewer than 5 diagnoses are likely)	Diagnostic Work-up: List immediate plans (up to 5) for further diagnostic work-up
1. Meningitis, bacterial	1. CT scan, brain
2. Meningitis, viral	2. Lumbar puncture with CSF analysis (opening pressure, antigen testing, gram stain, culture, protein and glucose levels)
3. Subarachnoid hemorrhage	3. CBC with differential
4. Vascular-type headache	4. Complete metabolic panel
5. Encephalitis	5.

1. Opening Scenario

James Patterson, a 23-year-old male, has come to the emergency room for evaluation of falling and fracturing his tooth.

2. Vital Signs

BP: 118/72 mmHg

Temp: 98.4° F (36.9° C)

HR: 54/minute, regular

RR: 12/minute

3. Examinee Tasks

1. Obtain a focused history.

2. Perform a relevant physical examination. (Do not perform breast, pelvic/genital, or rectal examination.)

3. Discuss your initial diagnostic impression and your work-up plan.

4. After leaving the room, complete your patient note on the given form.

Are the Vital Signs Stable?

Subjective

Knock, enter. Introduce yourself and place the first signpost.

"Hi Mr. Patterson, I'm Dr. Drake. I understand you had a fall today and broke a tooth? Can I ask you to explain what happened?"

"Yeah, doc. I was **running up the stairs** and **tripped**. I guess I fell and hit my face and broke my tooth. It was just an accident. I was just going too fast. Honestly, it wasn't a big deal, I was just…nothing."

"You sound a little hesitant. Do you recall the incident well?"

"Well, I kind of **blacked out**. It just happened and I **woke up,** and my tooth and lip hurt really bad. I could feel the sharp part of the tooth I broke. Actually, it was kind of freaky. Anyway, it's just an accident."

"Ok. So, did you lose consciousness?"

"**Yeah**, I guess I blacked out for a second. I was **heading up the stairs** and remember **waking up on the top stair** and my face hurt real bad. My friend was with me. He said I was just going up the stairs, and the next thing he knew, I was out. I think it was, you know, when you get up too fast and you're lightheaded? I just blacked out for a second. It was just an accident."

"When did this happen?"

"Maybe, a half-hour ago. Maybe 45 minutes, we came right here afterward."

"Alright. Did your friend say you shook when you were on the ground? Something like a seizure?"

"I **never asked** him. He said he just kept going up the stairs 'cause he didn't know I fell. I was behind him when it happened. He came back down **seconds later,** and I was just coming to. I remember him coming down and waking me up."

"Were you bleeding at all?"

"There was some blood, **yeah**. I **cut my lip** too. So we went inside my apartment and got a paper towel and held it on the cut. It was a small cut, but it bled pretty good for the size it was."

"Yeah, when you cut your face it can sure bleed a lot. Go back to the actual incident for me, if you would. Do you remember tripping on a stair then hitting your face, or did you pass out first and then fall?"

"I have **no idea**. I just was going up the stairs and the next thing I know, I was **waking up** and in pain. I was **really groggy**, too."

"Did your friend say how long you were unconscious?"

"No, but he had just turned around when he got to my apartment and looked and I wasn't there. I remember him sort of picking me up asking what happened. It must have been just **seconds**."

"Just before you passed out, did you have any chest pain or feeling like your heart was pounding?"

"**No**, nothing."

"How about dizziness or lightheadedness?"

"Well, I live on the third floor, and I have a habit of running up the stairs instead of walking. I **don't** get dizzy or anything, though."

"Has this ever happened to you before?"

"Passing out? Well, in college there were a few times I drank enough beer to pass out but never like this."

"Ok. Have you ever had a seizure?"

"**No**, not that I know of."

"How about any heart problems?"

"Again, **not that I know of**. I run track for my university so I'm pretty athletic, you know. I've been through a lot of sports physicals in the past, and no one's ever said anything like that."

"Have you ever had an ECG, or has a doctor ever looked at your heart with an ultrasound machine? Those are some tests that look for problems with the

---

Often a history obtained by a patient that can't be a direct witness is unreliable and choppy.

Attempting to determine if loss of consciousness occurred before a fall or because of a fall is important.

When a patient admits to excessive alcohol use, it may not be pertinent to go into the history of consumption at that part of the interview. Instead, make note of it, and revisit the subject later in the interview.

When asking about any medical test, make sure the patient knows exactly what the test is by explaining it briefly.

heart. An ECG is a test of the electrical activity of your heart and involves putting some sticky pads on your chest; you might remember that. The ultrasound machine might have been done to actually look at your heart beating."

"Oh, **no**, never."

"Ok. What was it you were doing before you had this incident?"

"My friend and I just got back from **playing racquetball**. We play on Mondays and Thursdays."

"Was there anything overtly strenuous about this workout?"

"**No**, it was the same as we always play. No difference really."

"Alright. Have you had any recent illnesses? Any minor health problems?"

"**No**, my last cold was maybe 3 months ago in the spring."

"How about nausea, vomiting, stomachaches, diarrhea?"

"Now that you mention it, I have had some **diarrhea** lately. I guess I forgot about that, it hasn't been a lot but just the **last few days**."

"Have you had any nausea or vomiting with that?"

"**Nah**, just the diarrhea. It's not explosive or anything, just loose and runny. That's why I forgot to mention it."

"Has there been any blood in the toilet or on the toilet paper when you're wiping?"

"**No**, not at all."

"Alright. How about any chest pain or feeling of pounding in your chest when you're not exercising?"

"**No**, my chest is fine. I don't feel like there's anything wrong with it."

"Alright. Are you on any medications?"

"**No**, I don't take anything."

"How about diet supplements?"

"I take **protein powder** in the morning. Its body-building protein."

"Are there any ingredients in it other than protein?"

"No, its **soy protein**, I'm sure about what's in it."

"Alright. Do you smoke or use other tobacco?"

"**No**, I'm in too many sports for that."

"You mentioned you drank beer before. Do you still?"

"**Yeah**."

"How much alcohol of any kind do you drink?"

"Well, I have a **few drinks in the week** but mainly on the weekends. I don't know, I go to the bars and have fun with my friends. I mean, I don't drink just to get drunk like I used to."

"How many drinks per night on the weekends would you say?"

"About **three or four** when I go out."

"When was the last time you drank?"

"Well, it's Thursday and I drank about three beers on Saturday night, so about **5 days**."

"Have you ever tried to cut down?"

"**No**, I don't think it's a problem."

"Have you ever felt annoyed by anyone talking about how much you drink?"

"**No**."

"Have you ever felt guilty about your drinking?"

"**No**."

"Have you ever had an eye opener in the morning? A drink to help wake you up or stave off a hangover?"

"**No**, I don't drink at all in the mornings."

"Have you been to the doctor for anything but a minor illness in your life? Especially anything you've stayed the night in the hospital for?"

"**No**, I've been healthy. This is the first time I've been to the emergency room. I've never stayed in the hospital."

"How about any surgeries?"

"Nope."

"Does anyone in your family have any major diseases?"

"Well, my dad has **high blood pressure**. My mom has some **depression**. My little brother has **Down's syndrome**. Otherwise they're all healthy."

"Specifically, has anyone had a problem with passing out?"

"**No**, not at all."

"You said your father has high blood pressure, any other problems with his heart at all?"

"**Nope**, not that I know of."

Signpost for the Physical Exam

"Ok. I'd like to do a physical exam now, if you don't mind. Just let me **wash my hands**. It looks like your **vital signs are normal,** so please let me first look in your ears…"

Objective

Points for Every Exam:

- Wash hands.
- Comment on vital signs, even if normal.
- Tell the patient where you are going to examine and disrobe.
- Do not repeat painful maneuvers.

Physical Exam:

Perform a focused physical, by system, from the head down.

System	Exam elements	Findings in this patient
Vitals	Check BP in each arm, noting differences aloud.	120/72 Right 118/70 Left
HEENT	Head: Examine the head for areas of trauma or swelling. Ears: Check the TMs visually and with an insufflator bulb. Eye: Check light reflexes bilaterally. Oral cavity: Examine the teeth and gums thoroughly, noting any abnormalities aloud. Check all rows of teeth for trauma. Inspect labial surfaces inside and out.	Head: atraumatic, normocephalic. Ears: pearly gray TMs bilaterally. Eyes: PERRLA. Mouth: right superior incisor break. No embedded fragments. Superior labial laceration to inside surface. Minimal bleeding. +Swelling, erythema, tenderness.
Neuro	Test tactile sensation of all four extremities and digital proprioception. Test motor strength of the extremities. Assess cranial nerves, deep tendon reflexes, sharp/dull testing, and dysdiadochokinesis. Perform gait assessment including heel- and toe-walks. Perform Romberg's testing for balance. Check Babinski's sign and ankle clonus.	Tactile sensation normal. Motor 5/5 throughout, CNs II–XII intact. Proprioception intact, dysdiadochokinesis normal, gait normal. DTRs 2+ and symmetric. Romberg negative. Babinski's downgoing. One beat of clonus.
Heart	Listen to four different auscultation areas on chest. Listen for carotid bruit's. Check pulses.	Regular rate/rhythm. No murmurs, rubs, or gallops.

Continue to gather information as you do the physical exam. Ask about pertinent aspects of each system as you perform the exams. Comment aloud on any real or simulated abnormalities.

Example: *"When you close your eyes, do you feel like you're going to fall?"*

Example: *"Do you have any pain in your ears?"*

End of Case

End by explaining you have several ideas of what could be wrong and could cause these symptoms. Tell the patient the first two diagnoses on your differential list and the major tests you'd now like to perform.

Example: *"Mr. Patterson, you've had what we call 'syncope,' which simple means an episode of passing out. Based on your account of the incident and your physical exam, I can't tell for sure what caused it. However, because that's a very important question to find the answer to, I'd like to run some tests on you. One reason for syncope is something called 'orthostatic hypotension.' This is caused when your body, for one reason or another, doesn't properly compensate for the normal drop in blood pressure that happens when we stand up or do a strenuous activity. We can test for this by checking your blood pressure in several different positions. Another possibility is that you had an abnormal heart rhythm, maybe just for a second, that caused a lack of oxygen to be delivered to your brain. For that possibility, I'd like to get an ECG, which is that test I'd talked about earlier to check the electrical activity of your heart. As well as these, I'd also like to get some blood work and a CT scan of your head. The CT scan is a special X-ray that can show cross-sections of your brain to show if there's any real damage done from this fall. As soon as I get the results, I'll be back in to discuss them with you. I'd like to step out now and arrange these with my nurse.*

Is there any other aspect of your health care we haven't already discussed? Ok then, thank you."

PATIENT NOTE

History: Include significant positives and negatives from history of present illness, past medical history, review of system(s), social history, and family history.

HPI: 23 y/o male with syncopal event a/w tooth fracture/facial trauma. Pt states he was running up stairs after a workout when LOC occurred, causing a fall onto stairs and causing tooth fracture and minor facial trauma. Unclear if LOC was before or after trauma. No direct witness of event although "seconds" afterward, witness able to help patient. Witnessed duration of LOC equal to seconds. No accompanying chest pain, palpitations, confusion, or dizziness before event. Question of postictal state although no witnessed convulsions. Patient admits to mild diarrhea x 2 days. Denies hematochezia.

Meds: None.

PMH: Recent mild diarrheal illness.

PSH: None.

Smoking: Denies.

Alcohol use: Socially. CAGE 0/4

FamH: Noncontributory.

Physical Examination: Indicate only pertinent positive and negative findings related to the patient's chief complaint.

VS Stable, normal. 120/72 Right, 118/70 Left.

HEENT: Head: Atraumatic, normocephalic. Ears: pearly gray TMs bilaterally. Eyes: PERRLA. Mouth: Right superior incisor fracture. No embedded fragments. Superior labial laceration to inside surface approximately 1 cm in length x 0.5 cm deep. Minimal bleeding. +Swelling, erythema, and ttp.

Neuro: Tactile sensation normal. Motor 5/5 and symmetric, CN's II-XII intact. Proprioception intact, dysdiadochokinesis normal, unassisted gait normal. DTR's 2+ and symmetric. Romberg's negative. Babinski's sign downgoing. One beat of clonus bilaterally.

Heart: RRR no murmurs, rubs, gallops. Pulse's normal. No carotid bruit's.

Differential Diagnosis: In order of likelihood (with 1 being the most likely), list up to 5 potential or possible diagnoses for this patient's presentation (in many cases, fewer than 5 diagnoses are likely)	Diagnostic Work-up: List immediate plans (up to 5) for further diagnostic work-up
1. Orthostatic hypotension	1. Orthostatic hypotension blood pressure measurements (tilt table testing).
2. Cardiac arrhythmia	2. CT scan, head
3. Vasovagal syncope	3. ECG
4. Idiopathic hypertrophic subaortic stenosis	4. CBC
5. Seizure	5. Complete metabolic panel

1. Opening Scenario

James Jackson, a 50-year-old male, has been admitted to the hospital, where he is seen for the first time for acute renal failure after presenting to the ER overnight. He has had an initial set of orders placed by the ER staff and the labs shown below.

Labs

Na:	138 mEq/L
K:	4.2 mEq/L
HCO3:	25 mEq/L
Cl:	100 mEq/L
BUN:	39 mg/dL
Creatinine:	3.0 mg/dL
Glucose:	103 mg/dL
CBC:	Normal

2. Vital Signs

BP:	130/86 mmHg
Temp:	98.9° F (37.2° C)
HR:	68/minute, regular
RR:	12/minute

3. Examinee Tasks

1. Obtain a focused history.

2. Perform a relevant physical examination. (Do not perform breast, pelvic/genital, or rectal examination.)

3. Discuss your initial diagnostic impression and your work-up plan.

4. After leaving the room, complete your patient note on the given form.

Are the Vital Signs Stable?

Subjective

Knock; enter. Introduce yourself, and place the first signpost.

"Hello, Mr. Jackson, I'm Dr. Schemple. I've reviewed your medical record and understand you've come into the hospital for kidney problems. I'd like to get the history of all this directly from you if you don't mind, so I can be clear on all that is going on. Can you start with what brought you to the emergency room?"

"Hi Dr. Schemple. I can tell you the story from the top. I'm a **construction worker**, chief supervisor in charge of concrete pouring for my company. Anyway, about **2 days ago** I was on the job and it was really **hot**, maybe 100 degrees. Well, I don't think I was drinking enough and I just got caught up in what I was doing and got **overheated**. I got to feeling really **dizzy** and **nauseated** all of a sudden. I drank some water and sat in the air conditioning a while and felt better. I drank a lot of flavored water, and by then it was time to go home. It was, like, maybe 45 minutes or something. That night, I didn't feel much like eating and felt sort of **nauseated and tired**. The next morning I got up and felt the same way and really sore—kind of like when you work out too much…and it really never went away since. So, as usual, I took some ibuprofen and went to work. It's sort of **been the same** over the last few days. I just haven't felt myself and am feeling really **weak**. So, I came into the emergency room after work."

"That sounds like a heck of a few days. Did you pass out at all during this episode?"

"**No**, I just got really **dizzy** and felt **nauseated,** and for a minute, I **didn't know where I was…kind of confused**. It was weird."

"I'll bet that was strange. Have you ever passed out or had this type of feeling when you were in the heat before?"

"**No**, not in 27 years working outside. I just got **overheated**; I've seen it a thousand times. It's not that big of a deal; it's just that I **never felt right again**."

"Ok. Let me ask a little about the episode. What happened when you felt dizzy?"

"Well, I told the guys, because we were pouring a foundation at the time, I was going to go sit down. I went to the side of the truck and sat down. That helped a little, but I was so hot I got into the cab then and turned the **air conditioning on**. I mean, I was thinking 'What would I tell one of my workers to do in that situation? Ya know? So I got in the air conditioning."

"What was the activity you were doing at the time?"

"I had been out pouring a foundation. I'd been out there about **2 hours,** and, you know, it was around 100 degrees that day. I was **sweating** a lot and just forgot to **drink water**."

"Were you standing up in the sun or sitting?"

One of the hallmarks of heat stroke is mental status change (which may or may not involve LOC)

"I was **standing** and guiding the pour. That's my job."

"Ok. Do you remember having chest pain or palpitations?"

"**No**, none of that."

"Ok. As I understand it, after the incident you went home. Did you still have the feeling of dizziness?"

"**Yeah**, for the rest of that night, I did. Then I got up in the morning and went to work and felt it. It's just hasn't gotten better."

"You said you took some ibuprofen as well. How much have you taken since the incident?"

"I took a few, maybe **six since the whole thing happened**. It's the **prescription strength** ones I get from my doctor when I have trouble with my **gout**. I think they're **800 milligrams**."

"Ok. Did that help?"

"**Not at all**, it didn't touch it."

"Do you normally take ibuprofen?"

"**Yeah**, most days."

"How much do you take?"

"Oh, about **two a day**. I have **joint pains** from all those years of working outside. My **gout** also makes things hard. My doctor said it's ok to take when my gout flares up."

"For how long have you been taking it at that dose?"

"Oh, I've taken it for a good **5 years now**. It's been since I got diagnosed with gout about then."

"Alright. Did you take any other medicines?"

"**Not for this**; I'm just on my other medicine for gout, **allopurinol**. I take a blood pressure medicine, too."

"What's the name of that blood pressure medicine?"

"It's called **H-C-T-Z**. I can't pronounce the whole name. I take it once in the morning."

"Ok. I know what that is. Do you take any other medicines?"

"**No**, that's enough, doc."

"Alright. So to go back to what happened if you would, was there an event that brought you to the emergency room last night, or was it just the overall feeling you described that wasn't going away?"

"It was that **feeling**. **Nausea** and that **'out-of-sorts'**-type feeling. I put in my day at work and didn't have time to make an appointment at my doctor's. I can't take time off, but I figured I should come get checked out. So, I came into the ER, and the doctor said I had problems enough with my kidneys that I had to come stay the night. He **explained the test results** and showed me what was wrong. That was about 3:00 in the morning so it wasn't very long ago, actually."

"Yeah, sometimes the emergency room can be quite a wait. Did you get any sleep last night?"

"**Not much**, but, you know, this is more important so I don't mind."

> Never admonish a patient for not following medication instructions or taking a medication incorrectly, especially during the interview phase.

> Transition statement of empathy

"Do you feel like you understand the test results and what they mean?"

"Yeah, the emergency room doc was very nice about it. **He explained** all about how the kidneys sometimes don't work right and those labs, the **BUN** and **creatinine,** show it. I feel like I know what's going on."

"Great. If you feel like you want me to review with you, please feel free to ask. I certainly appreciate your patience. Well, let me ask a little bit more about your medical history. You mentioned you had gout and high blood pressure. I understand the medicines you're taking. Are there any other diseases or illnesses you've seen the doctor for?"

"**No**, that's enough if you ask me."

"When was the last time you had a gouty flare-up, and where was it?"

"Oh, about **6 months ago**. I had it in my **toe** on my **right foot**. That's usually where I have it."

"Alright, thinking about your urine lately, has it appeared unusual in any way?"

"Yeah, it's been **really dark**, actually. Like a **deep orange**."

"Has there been any blood in it?"

"**No** blood I think, but just dark. Didn't look red but maybe it was dark from that, I don't know."

"Have you had other problems, like burning or pain when you urinate?"

"**No**, never have."

"How about going to the bathroom a lot lately or especially at night?"

"**No**, not really. In fact, it seems like I've **slowed down** over the last **few days**."

"Ok. Have you felt like you have to go and couldn't, or have you just not needed to go?"

"I just **haven't needed to go**. That's another reason I'm trying to drink more."

"Do you ever feel like it's hard to start a stream or that when you do go, it's hard to empty all the way out?"

"**No**, I don't feel like that."

"Ok. Have you ever had any surgeries?"

"**No**, I've been lucky."

"Ok. Do you smoke or use tobacco products?"

"I **quit smoking** about **3 years ago**. I smoked for about **20 years**, though. My doctor helped me with that."

"Well, that's great. How about drinking alcohol?"

"**Yeah**, I drink about **a beer or two a day**. After work I just can't give up my beer."

"Do you drink more on the weekends?"

"**No**, that's about it."

"Have you ever tried to cut down?"

"**No**, not really."

"Have you ever felt annoyed by someone talking about your alcohol intake?"

Asking if the patient understands the current medical situation or the ER course can strengthen your relationship.

In renal failure, group major diagnoses into three main categories:
 Pre-renal
 Renal
 Post-renal

"**Yeah,** my wife sometimes, but my drinking isn't the only thing she annoys me about."

"Do you ever feel guilty because of your drinking?"

"**No**."

"Have you ever woken up and had a drink in the morning as an 'eye opener?'"

"**No**, never done that."

"Ok. Do take any other drugs, for recreation, I mean?"

"**No**, I used to smoke some **pot,** but that was **decades ago**."

"Alright. How about any health issues in your family? Has anyone related to you had a serious health problem?"

"My dad had **kidney stones** before he died. He died of a **heart attack** at age **77**. My mom's still alive and has **emphysema** from smoking all her life. That's one of the reasons I quit. Otherwise, my little brother's healthy."

Signpost for the Physical Exam

"Ok. I'd like to do a physical exam now, if you don't mind. Just let me **wash my hands**. First I'd like to examine your ears…"

Objective

Points for Every Exam:

- Wash hands.
- Comment on vital signs, even if normal.
- Tell the patient where you are going to examine and disrobe.
- Do not repeat painful maneuvers.

Physical Exam:

Perform a focused physical, by system, from the head down.

System	Exam elements	Findings in this patient
HEENT	Examine the ears with an insufflator bulb and otoscope. Eyes: Examine reactivity with an ophthalmoscope, then proceed with retinal exam. Make sure to focus on the optic disc and make a comment about blurring of the optic disc. Examine the nose and throat briefly. Check for nystagmus.	Normal findings. Normal TMs. PERLA, No blurring of the optic disc. No nystagmus
Neurologic	Complete a cranial nerve exam, Babinski's, Romberg's, and finger-to-nose tests. Assess the tactile sense of all extremities along with proprioception and sharp/dull testing. Perform deep tendon reflexes, motor strength, and dysdiadochokinesis. Observe the patient's gait including heel-walk and toe-walk.	Normal neurologic exam. CNs II–XII intact, Romberg's test, finger-to-nose, and Babinski's test normal. Symmetric DTRs, tactile sense, sharp/dull testing normal. Motor strength 5/5 and symmetric, gait normal, Romberg's test normal. Dysdiadochokinesis normal.

Abdomen	Percuss the costovertebral angle (CVA) for pain. Listen for bowel sounds and abdominal bruit's. Gently palpate all four quadrants and the epigastrim, noting any tenderness or masses.	Normal BS's. No ttp, including over the epigastrim. No masses. No abdominal bruit's. No CVA tenderness.

Continue to gather information as you do the physical exam. Comment aloud on any real or simulated abnormalities.

Example: *"Do you have any pain when I strike here? [while percussing the CVA's]"*

Example: *"Does it hurt when I press here? [while applying direct pressure of the bladder region]"*

End of Case

End by explaining you have several ideas of what could be wrong and could cause these symptoms. Tell the patient the first two diagnoses on your differential list and the major tests you'd now like to perform.

Example: *"Mr. Jackson, you were admitted for what is called renal failure, which you certainly have by the testing that was taken when you were admitted to the hospital. The question is 'Why?' From talking with you and doing a physical exam, there are several possibilities that I'd like to run some tests for. First, you very well may have had a serious heat injury a few days ago. That can damage several organs in your body, including your kidneys. Because it has been some time since the incident itself, it may be hard to actually determine if that was the initial problem, but nonetheless, I'd like to get some blood work to answer that question. Also, this could be from interactions between your medications, especially the amount and duration you've been taking of that ibuprofen. At that dose, and over time, it can harm the kidneys and cause some damage that you might not have noticed until now. I would also like to examine your blood for that possibility. As well, as those problems I mentioned, I'd also like to do a prostate exam on you today to check the size of your prostate. Sometimes, men your age can have a slowly enlarging prostate gland that can actually contribute to kidney damage and problems urinating. Despite you reporting no problems with urination, I'd like to do this simple exam to check for enlargement. I'll step out for a few minutes and arrange these tests with the nurse and ask for an escort during this exam.*
Is there any other aspect of your health care we haven't already discussed? Ok then, thank you."

PATIENT NOTE

History: Include significant positives and negatives from history of present illness, past medical history, review of system(s), social history, and family history.

HPI: 50 y/o male admitted to the hospital for acute renal failure. Pt has significant history of possible heat injury 2 days prior to admission causing persistent symptoms of nausea, muscle aches, and mental status change felt as an "out-of-sorts" feeling. He denies LOC but endorses the beginning of these mental status symptoms in conjunction with his recent heat event. He removed himself from the environment, drank fluids, and then went home. Throughout the subsequent days symptoms remained despite self-medication with ibuprofen 800 mg x six. He endorses dark urine but denies overt blood, dysuria, or frequency. He also denies weak urinary stream, incomplete voiding, nocturia. History also is pertinent for use of ibuprofen, 1600 mg/day for about 5 years.

PMH: Gout—treated; hypertension—treated.

PSH: None.

Tobacco: Twenty pack-years. Quit x 3 yrs.

EtOH: 1-2 beers/day. No increase on weekends. CAGE 1/4, negative.

Drugs: Denies.

Meds: Allopurinol, HCTZ, ibuprofen 800 mg bid (increased to 3 per day over last 2 days).

FamH: Father—urolithiasis, deceased age 77 from MI; mother—emphysema.

Physical Examination: Indicate only pertinent positive and negative findings related to the patient's chief complaint.

VS Stable.

HEENT: Normal TMs. PERLA, No blurring of the optic disc. No nystagmus.

Neurologic: CNs II–XII intact, finger-to-nose, and Babinski's test normal. Symmetric DTR's. Tactile sense, sharp/dull testing normal. Motor strength 5/5 and symmetric. Gait normal, Romberg's test normal. Dysdiadochokinesis normal.

Abdomen: No TTP. No masses. Normal BSs. No abdominal bruit's. No CVA tenderness. No hepatosplenomegally.

Differential Diagnosis: In order of likelihood (with 1 being the most likely), list up to 5 potential or possible diagnoses for this patient's presentation (in many cases, fewer than 5 diagnoses are likely)	Diagnostic Work-up: List immediate plans (up to 5) for further diagnostic work-up.
1. Heat stroke causing nephrotoxicity	1. Urine analysis with urine myoglobin and culture
2. NSAID-induced glomerulonephritis	2. Urine creatinine, urine sodium, plasma creatinine, plasma sodium (calculate FENa)
3. Dehydration-induced renal failure	3. Ionized Ca, phosphate, uric acid, CPK level, and liver function panel with transaminases.
4. Glomerulonephritis	4. ECG
5. Cerebellar stroke	5. MRI brain

1. Opening Scenario

Janis Clark, a 42-year-old Caucasian female, presents with complaints of feeling a lump in her left breast.

2. Vital Signs

BP: 128/66 mmHg

Temp: 98.6° F (37° C)

HR: 56/minute, regular

RR: 16/minute

3. Examinee Tasks

1. Obtain a focused history.

2. Perform a relevant physical examination. (Do not perform breast, pelvic/genital, or rectal examination.)

3. Discuss your initial diagnostic impression and your work-up plan.

4. After leaving the room, complete your patient note on the given form.

Are the Vital Signs Stable?

Subjective

Knock; enter. Introduce yourself, and place the first signpost.

"Hello, Ms. Clark, I'm Dr. Semelis. I understand you've recently found a troubling mass in your breast. Please tell me more about it?"

"Yes doctor, I found a **lump in the left one** about a **week ago** and wanted to come in right away because my **sister-in-law** also had breast cancer and she's getting treatment right now. I was in the shower and decided to do a breast exam, you know. I don't know if I was doing it right, but I've done it this way a few times. I think I feel a breast lump right here [indicating the **superior lateral quadrant** of the left breast]. I just don't want to find out I have breast cancer, too. Do you think that's what it could be?"

"Well, it's a good thing you came in because I find it best to evaluate all breast lumps right away for the possibility of cancer. I understand it can be unnerving

Significant health events occurring to those around the patient often lead to fear and worry.

Address patient concerns such as cancer as soon as the patient brings them up. Don't discount their fears, but inform on the next steps in diagnosis.

to find a lump in your breast. However, keep in mind, cancer is just one thing that may cause breast lumps. Sometimes it's what we call 'benign breast disease' rather than cancer, which would be good news. The possibility of breast cancer is real, however, so I'd like to examine you myself in a few minutes. First let me gather a bit more information, ok? Does the lump feel painful?"

"No, it's **not painful**, but it seems like I'm constantly rubbing the spot."

"Have you ever felt this lump before?"

"This is the first time I actually found anything in the shower. I've done exams before. Not every month like I'm supposed to, but it's whenever I can remember."

"Have you ever been shown how to do a breast self-exam?"

"Well, **no**. My doctor did one on me once and said I can do them on myself. I got a pamphlet on it, but think I lost it. I just tried to do what he did before."

"Ok. Tell me where in your menstrual cycle you are now."

"My period ended **about 3 weeks ago**, now. I'm on the **pill**, I've been on it for a long time, you know. I'm pretty regular."

"Is that a combination hormone pill?"

"Yeah, it's called **ortho novum**."

"Ok. So may I understand you have a regular period every month?"

"Yeah, I'm pretty **regular.**"

"Does this lump change in relation to your period?"

"I **don't know** if it makes a difference when I'm on a different part of my period. I haven't waited long enough to know if it's still there during other parts of my cycle."

"Alright. Have you had any unusual changes in your skin over the lump itself or any unusual nipple discharge?"

"**No,** I haven't. Like I said, it might be a little sore from me pressing on it so much."

"Is this the first breast lump you've ever felt in either breast?"

"Thank god, **yes**."

"I know you said it might be a little sore from you pressing on it, but does it feel tender right now?"

"Nah, not really. I mean, it doesn't really hurt. Maybe it's because I just know it's there. It's not painful or anything."

"How large would you say it is? That is, would you compare it to a pea, a peanut, a walnut, or any other type of object?"

"Umm. Maybe about **the size of a peanut** or so. Yeah, about a peanut."

"And has the skin ever been sore or red around it?"

"**No**, not really."

"Have you ever had a mammogram?"

"I **haven't,** although my doctor said I should. I was going to, but I went on vacation. He said I should schedule it after I got back, but I never got around to it. That was last year. I guess I should."

Often the patient will remember the brand name of the medication, which may tell you more than the patient can.

Risk Factors for Breast Cancer
- Age
- Caucasian race
- Benign breast disease with cytologic atypia
- Personal history of breast cancer
- Higher socioeconomic status
- Lack of physical activity
- High dietary fat intake
- Lifetime exposure to endogenous estrogens (influenced by age of menarche, parity, age of menopause, etc.)
- Family history and genetic factors
- Exposure to ionizing radiation

"A mammogram's a good screening test for women your age. We'll talk about that more depending on the results of this investigation. Let me ask about your family a little bit. You mentioned your sister-in-law having breast cancer. Is she related to you by blood?"

"**No,** she's my brother's wife. We've always been close, since teenagers. Her doctor found it in her 2 months ago. She got all the tests and found out it was cancer. She's scheduled for surgery next week. She's really scared about it. The doctors say it's really lucky she caught it so early, though."

"Has there been anyone in your direct family with any kind of cancer, especially breast?"

"My mom lives in Florida, and she had a **stroke** and was lucky to survive. She lives with my brother now. My dad has **prostate cancer,** I think. But they told him they wouldn't operate on it. They're just watching him, I guess. I also have a sister, and she's doing fine living up in Michigan. She's younger than me. My brother's fine, too."

"Have you had children or been pregnant in your life?"

"I've been pregnant **three times** but had a **miscarriage** in between my two boys. They're both healthy."

"Do you remember how old you were when you got your first period?"

"I was **14 years old**. I remember it really well because I hated it at first. I've been blessed with a fairly regular period my whole life though. I cramp somewhat, but the women in my family, other than me, all have worse periods than me. So I'm kind of lucky."

"Ok. Do you smoke or drink alcohol?"

"**No**, I've **never smoked**. I hate when my husband smokes cigars on his poker nights. I don't drink either."

"Do you exercise regularly?"

"**Not really**. I mean to, but all my exercise comes from chores like shopping or picking up my kids at baseball practice."

"Are you on any medications besides your birth control? Or are you allergic to anything?

"I was taking fish oil for awhile but quit that. I also take a headache medicine called **Maxalt** but only take that when I need to. Nothing else."

"Sounds like you have some migraine headaches. Are there any other problems you see the doctor for? Have you ever spent the night in the hospital?"

"Yeah, I have **migraines**. Otherwise, I **rarely see the doctor**. I've spent the night in the hospital with my two children. I lived in Texas at the time for both of them. I kind of avoid doctors and hospital and stuff if I can. No other problems."

"Have you ever had any other problems with breast disease in your life?"

"No, nothing."

"How about surgeries?"

"Well, I had a **C-section** with my second baby. He was breech. Nothing else, though."

Signpost for the Physical Exam

"Ok. I'd like to do a physical exam now, if you don't mind. Just let me wash my hands. It looks like your **vital signs are normal.** I'd like to ask you to remove your shirt so I may listen to your back and chest…" [For this exam, a mannequin will be provided for direct exam skills. Do not examine the patient.]

Objective

Points for Every Exam:

- Wash hands.
- Comment on vital signs, even if normal.
- Tell the patient where you are going to examine and disrobe.
- Do not repeat painful maneuvers.

Physical Exam:

Perform a focused physical, by system, from the head down.

System	Exam elements	Findings in this patient
Breast (Mannequin provided)	Drapes are provided, uncover only one breast at a time. Start with observation (make comment on symmetry or skin changes). Ask the patient to point out the area of the lump. In the supine position, start with the center and palpate in a spiraling manner using the pads of your fingers to feel any underlying density. After the main breast is done, palpate the superior lateral quadrant, axilla, supraclavicular area, and medial area of the arm. Alternatively, examine each half at a time, working from top to bottom with fingertips. Concentrate on the superior lateral quadrant. Palpate the axillary lymph node group. Then go back to concentrate on the area pointed out by the patient.	No skin changes noted in symmetric breasts. Notable lump in upper outer quadrant of left breast. No axillary or supraclavicular lymphadenopathy. No expressible nipple discharge.

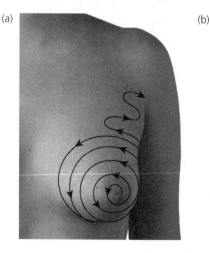
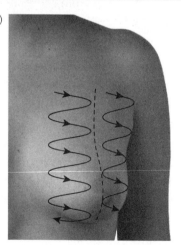

(a)   (b)

FIGURE 10.1 Two methods for the systematic palpation of the breast. (a) Work circumferentially from the areola. (b) Examine each half at a time, working from top to bottom.

Reprinted with permission from Thomas & Monahan. *Oxford Handbook of Clinical Examination and Practical Skills.* Oxford University Press, 2007.

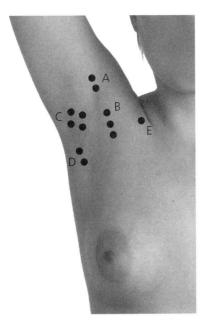

A = Lateral
B = Pectoral
C = Central
D = Subscapular
E = Infraclavicular

FIGURE 10.2 Axillary lymph nodes.

Reprinted with permission from Thomas & Monahan, *Oxford Handbook of Clinical Examination and Practical Skills*. Oxford University Press, 2007.

Continue to gather information as you do the physical exam. Comment aloud on any real or simulated abnormalities.

Example: *If you feel the lump: "Would you say this is as large as it has ever been?"*

Example: *"Have you had any nipple discharge lately?"*

End of Case

End by explaining you have several ideas of what could be wrong and could cause these symptoms. Tell the patient the first two diagnoses on your differential list and the major tests you'd now like to perform.

Example: *"Ms. Clark, there are several possibilities for the nature of this breast lump. Breast lumps can be caused, again, by 'benign breast disease' but can also be cancerous. Obviously, cancer, or what we call 'precancer,' is sometimes found in a breast lump and is the most important thing to diagnose early. I'd like to schedule you for further investigation of this lump. I'd like to do an ultrasound of the lump to better determine if it may be a fluid filled pocket, called a cyst, or a solid mass. However, we may need to move onto a biopsy. The best way to evaluate a lump in the breast that I can also feel is a biopsy. This type of biopsy is a minor surgery in which we take a very small needle and insert it into the lump itself. We can then look under a microscope for cancer cells. It means you'll have to be scheduled and come in for the procedure, but it's the best way to evaluate this. If the biopsy is negative, we can talk about further steps to do periodic screening and self-breast exams. If it's positive, we'll proceed with a treatment plan. Keep in mind, though, cancer is not the only thing that may cause a lump in your breast. Sometimes other benign processes cause this symptom, which we should be able to tell by the biopsy. I'd like to step out now and make arrangements for your biopsy.*

Is there any other aspect of your health care we haven't already discussed? Ok then, thank you."

PATIENT NOTE

History: Include significant positives and negatives from history of present illness, past medical history, review of system(s), social history, and family history.

HPI: 42 y/o Caucasian female c/o palpable breast lump discovered 1 week ago. She first felt this in the shower on a periodic breast exam done at approximately week 2 of her menstrual cycle. She states the lump is asymptomatic without notable change with menses. Size is reported as about consistent with a peanut, nonchanging, and not associated with skin changes or pain. Recent history of nonsanguinous relative with breast cancer. LMP approximately 3 wks ago.

OBHx: G3P2. Menarche age 14. Currently on combination OCP. No prior mammography.

PMH: Non contributory.

PSH: Cesarean section x 1.

Tobacco: Denies.

Alcohol use: Denies.

Meds: Ortho-Novum, Maxalt-PRN.

FamH: Mother—CVA; father-prostate cancer.

Physical Examination: Indicate only pertinent positive and negative findings related to the patient's chief complaint.

VS Stable.

Gen: Ill appearing, no acute distress.

Breast: Observation: normal symmetric breasts. No skin changes or nipple discharge noted. Positive palpable breast mass approx 1 cm diameter in upper outer quadrant. No ttp. No fluctuance, no erythema, no induration.

Differential Diagnosis: In order of likelihood (with 1 being the most likely), list up to 5 potential or possible diagnoses for this patient's presentation (in many cases, fewer than 5 diagnoses are likely)	Diagnostic Work-up: List immediate plans (up to 5) for further diagnostic work-up
1. Fibroadenoma	1. Breast ultrasound
2. Breast malignancy or carcinoma *in situ*	2. Needle core biopsy
3. Fibrocystic changes	3. CBC
4. Intraductal papilloma	4. Basic metabolic panel including electrolytes, renal function, and glucose
5. Mammary duct ectasia	5. Liver enzyme panel

11   Chest Pain

1. Opening Scenario

Andrea Torwell, a 37-year-old female, presents to the emergency department for evaluation of chest pain lasting 4 hours.

2. Vital Signs

BP:	154/90 mmHg
Temp:	99.0° F (37.2° C)
HR:	84/minute, regular
RR:	18/minute
Pulse oximetry:	100% on room air

3. Examinee Tasks

1. Obtain a focused history.

2. Perform a relevant physical examination. (Do not perform breast, pelvic/genital, or rectal examination.)

3. Discuss your initial diagnostic impression and your work-up plan.

4. After leaving the room, complete your patient note on the given form.

Are the Vital Signs Stable?

Subjective

Knock; enter. Introduce yourself, and place the first signpost.

"Hello Ms. Torwell, I'm Dr. Jessul. I understand you've been having some chest pain. Please tell me when this started."

"Yeah, doctor. It started about **4 hours** ago and **woke** me up from sleep. Am I having a heart attack?"

"Well, that's a good question I'd like to find the answer to as well. I see you're on oxygen and you've been given some nitroglycerin, morphine, and aspirin. These are all excellent medications to treat a heart attack, just in case you are having one. The first thing I want to do is talk to you briefly, then we'll

Patients may often jump to the most life-threatening possibility before the interview is complete. It's important to address these concerns up front and give a confident answer on the next step.

proceed with some important tests to determine what the cause of your pain is. Do you still have the pain?"

"It's **still there** in the left side a little. It used to be a lot worse, though."

"Can you tell me what it felt like when you woke up?"

"Yeah, it felt like a really severe pain in the **center of my chest**. Like I was being **stabbed** right there [pointing to the midsternum]. It was intense and made me sit right up in bed. At the time, I was **sweaty**, too. I went to the kitchen and drank some **milk**, because I thought it was something I ate, you know, but it just didn't help. So I got my husband up, and he said if I feel bad enough 'call an ambulance.' Well, I didn't call an ambulance, but he brought me here."

"Alright. Do you remember if the pain radiated down one of your arms or into your neck?"

"It sort of went into my arm for a while. My **left arm**, but then it stopped. Never into my neck. It's kind of scary. I don't want to have a heart attack. I…"

"I bet it is scary. I hope to help as we do all the testing necessary and treat you as fast as we can. I don't know if it is your heart because there are other things that might cause the same type of pain in your chest. We're working on finding all that out right away, ok?"

"Yeah."

"Ok. Did it make the arm numb, or was it only pain?"

"It was **pain**. Like the feeling in my **chest hurt so bad it was making my arm hurt**. Kind of **dull**, though, not that stabbing like in my chest."

"On a scale of 0 to 10, 10 being the worst pain imaginable, what number would you give this pain at its worst?"

"Oh, it was an **11**. It really hurt."

"And what number would you give it now?"

"I'd say more like a **1 or 2**. It hurts a lot less now after that medicine. I have a headache, though."

Explain expected medication side effects to the patient. Give them as much knowledge as possible about the pain they're having.

"Well, I'm glad there's such a difference. The headache sometimes happens from the medicine we give you initially. Please know it's necessary to prevent further damage if indeed this is a heart attack. Other than the medicine, were you able to decrease the pain on your own at all? Such as with a change in position?"

"It felt a **little better when I sat up**. It seems to be worse **when I lay down but not much**. That milk I drank when I woke up didn't do anything."

"How about any things you did that made the pain worse? Such as breathing deeply?"

"It was **worse when I took a deep breath**. When it hurt the worst I had to take these **short, fast breaths**. It hurt to fully **inhale**. Now [as she takes a large breath] it hurts when I really take a deep breath, too, but worse when breathing really, really deeply."

"Were there any other symptoms along with this? Such as coughing or lightheadedness?"

"**No**, I didn't have anything else. Other than the trouble breathing and pain. I didn't focus on much else."

"How about pain in other areas of your body? Especially in the lower parts of your legs?"

"Umm, **no**, nothing like that."

"You'd mentioned earlier you had been sweating in bed. How much were you sweating? Was this sweating through the sheets or just a little?"

"Well, I mean, I felt pretty wet when I woke up. I think it had only been around the time I woke up because the sheets weren't really wet. When I went to the kitchen I was shaking a little, too, because I was **afraid of having a heart attack**. My husband made a comment about me being all sweaty when he saw me though, so I guess I was."

"Ok. Have you had any recent illnesses?"

"No, I'm on a few medications from the doctor. But I haven't had the flu or anything lately."

"Have you recently had a fever?"

"**No.**"

"Ok. Please tell me about those illnesses you've had in the past. The ones your doctor is treating or any others."

"Yeah, well, I have something called **polycystic ovarian syndrome**. They call it PCOS. I take a drug called **Metformin** for that. I also have some depression that I take **Zoloft** for. I take my daily birth control, **orthotricyclin**, it's called. Then I've also been taking a drug called **Wellbutrin** to try to quit smoking. I feel like I take a lot of pills."

"You certainly seem to be on a few. I bet it's hard to remember all of those."

"Well, I do it. Most of them are in the morning anyway. Then at night."

"Are there any other problems in your past medical history you've seen the doctor for? Especially requiring you to stay the night in the hospital?"

"I was in here with the **delivery of my daughter**. She's 7 years old now. Otherwise, I've never been in the hospital."

"Have you ever had chest pain before?"

"I have some **heart burn** from time to time. Who doesn't? But it doesn't feel like this really. I take **Tums** or another **antacid,** and it helps a little. I have a sensitive stomach overall."

"Is this the only time you've felt this type of pain and this severe?"

"Oh, yeah. **Definitely**."

"Have you had any vomiting or nausea with this?"

"**No**, not at all."

"How about any belly pain or diarrhea lately?"

"**No**, I had that **heartburn**, like I mentioned, about **2 nights ago**, but no diarrhea."

"Ok. Any other problems such as vision changes or numbness?"

"**No**, none of that."

It's always best to ask about general allergies rather than only drug allergies.

"Alright. Have you had any surgeries?"

"**No**, never."

"Ok. How about any allergies? Are you allergic to anything?"

"**Carrots** make me break out if I eat a lot of them. Nothing else though."

"I understand you smoke. Is that cigarettes? And how much?"

"Yeah, I know I should quit. It's **cigarettes**. I smoke about **half a pack per day**. I cut down though, I used to smoke much more. I'm quitting, you know."

"How much did you smoke before? And for how long?"

"Oh, I've smoked for **10 years**. It was about a pack per day for that. My husband convinced me to get on this new medicine. I started it about 3 weeks ago. I cut down since then."

"Ok. How about drinking alcohol?"

"I have a **glass of wine** or so at a party or barbeque. I don't drink much more than that. Maybe two glasses on New Year's."

"Do you take any other drugs? Especially such as IV drugs?"

"Oh **no**. Never have."

"Ok. How about your family's health issues? Does anyone in your family have heart disease?"

"My **mom** has had **two heart attacks**. She was **54** years old the first time, and it happened then again when she was **59 years old**. She survived both of them, but now she's on a very strict diet and stuff. My **dad** has **high blood pressure,** but that's all. He works out all the time and is pretty healthy. I'm an only child so I don't have brothers and sisters. My kids are very healthy."

"Do you get any regular exercise?"

"I do my exercise videos. At least I try. It's kind of hard for me because of work. I do them about **twice per week**. I should get more."

Signpost for the Physical Exam

"Ok. I'd like to do a physical exam now, if you don't mind. Just let me **wash my hands.** The first think I'd like to examine is your heart. Please allow me to put my stethoscope inside your gown to listen…"

Objective

Points for Every Exam:

- Wash hands.
- Comment on vital signs, even if normal.
- Tell the patient where you are going to examine and disrobe.
- Do not repeat painful maneuvers.

Physical Exam:

Perform a focused physical, by system, from the head down.

System	Exam elements	Findings in this patient
Neck	Check for asymmetry or lymphadenopathy. When the patient is reclining (at any angle), check for JVD by both direct observation and tangential light observation. Check the carotid pulse and listen for bruit's.	No lymphadenopathy. No JVD. Normal carotid pulse and no bruit's.
Heart	Listen for heart sounds in at least four different auscultation points. Feel for the point of maximal impulse (PMI). While auscltating the heart, feel radial and peripheral pulses. Check capillary refill.	RRR no murmurs/rubs/gallops. Peripheral pulses 2+ bilaterally. Cap refill <2 secs. BP normal.
Lungs	Auscultate the posterior and lateral lung fields. Make sure to listen to 6 points on the posterior lung fields and 1 on each lateral lung field.	Clear to auscultation. No rhonchi, rubs, or rales.
Abdomen	Listen for bowel sounds. Gently palpate all four quadrants and the epigastrim. Check Murphy's sign. Check for rebound tenderness over McBurney's point.	Normal BSs. No ttp, including over epigastrim. No masses.
Extremities	Examine the lower extremities, including the thighs and calves. Palpate for tenderness, swelling, induration, or fluctuance bilaterally. Observe for symmetry. Check Homan's sign.	Normal exam of both lower extremities. No swelling, tenderness, erythema. Negative Homan's sign.

Continue to gather information as you do the physical exam. Comment aloud on any real or simulated abnormalities.

Example: *"Please take a long inhalation for me while I listen to your lungs."*

Example: *"Does it hurt when I press firmly here?* [while applying direct pressure to the epigastrim]*"*

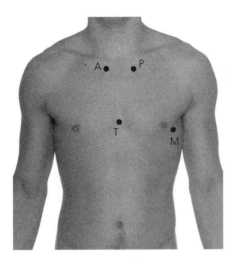

A = Aortic
P = Pulmonary
T = Tricuspid
M = Mitral

FIGURE 11.1 The four standard areas for auscultation of the precordium and the valves that are best heard at each area.

Reprinted with permission from Thomas & Monahan. *Oxford Handbook of Clinical Examination and Practical Skills.* Oxford University Press, 2007.

TABLE 11.1 Electrocardiogram Changes With Time Following Myocardial Infarction.

Within hours	T waves	Abnormally tall
Within hours	ST segments	Rise above the baseline
Less than 24 h	T waves	Inverted
Less than 24 h	ST segments	Return to baseline
Within days	Pathological Q waves	Present
Later	T waves	May or may not remain inverted
Later	Pathological Q waves	May persist

Reprinted with permission from Cox & Roper. Clinical Skills. Oxford University Press, 2005.

End of Case

End by explaining you have several ideas of what could be wrong and could cause these symptoms. Tell the patient the first two diagnoses on your differential list and the major tests you'd now like to perform.

Example: *"Ms. Torwell, it's a good thing you've come into the hospital today because chest pain can be a sign of something serious. I can't say if you're having a heart attack right now, but that's one of my main concerns to investigate first. I'd like to look into this with several tests, including blood work and an ECG, which takes an electrical picture of how your heart's beating. There are other critical things in your chest that may be causing this pain as well, namely your lungs. So for those, I'd also like to get some blood work and an X-ray. Also, I'd like to obtain a CT scan, or "Cat Scan" of your chest since sometimes chest pain can be caused by a blood clot in the lungs. Considering your risk factors of being on birth control medicines and smoking, this could be a possibility. Depending on the results, there might be some additional tests that need to be ordered afterward. Besides these most important issues, chest pain may also be caused by structures that won't threaten your life, such as your chest wall, the muscles and bones, or your esophagus. It's hard to tell until we get the results of your tests. I'd like to step out now and arrange for these to be completed.*

Is there any other aspect of your health care we haven't already discussed? Ok then, thank you."

PATIENT NOTE

History: Include significant positives and negatives from history of present illness, past medical history, review of system(s), social history, and family history.

HPI: 37 y/o female with midsternal chest pain x 4 hours. Pain sharp and stabbing with peak intensity at 11/10 and current level 1–2/10 after medications. Onset of pain during sleep and reported as waking the patient up. Pt on oxygen at time of interview and s/p Morphine, Aspirin, and Nitroglycerin. Pt states pleuritic component, especially when intensity was worst, but only now when on deep inhalation. Questionable worsening of pain on laying down, no apparent association with exertion. Diaphoresis noted with symptom onset. Positive h/o reflux although these symptoms differ in character/intensity.

ROS: No n/v/d, last episode reflux 2 days ago. No lower extremity pain. No fever, lightheadedness, or mental status change. O/w noncontributory.

PMH: G1P1, PCOS-treated, depression-treated, GERD-treated OTC.

PSH: None.

Tobacco: ½ ppd currently, 10 pack-years. Current treatment of Bupropion.

EtOH: Socially, rare.

Drugs: Denies.

Meds: Metformin, Wellbutrin, Ortho-tricyclen, Zoloft, and OTC antacids.

FamH: Mother—two MIs, age 54, 59 years; father—hypertension.

Physical Examination: Indicate only pertinent positive and negative findings related to the patient's chief complaint.

VS Stable.

Neck: Negative JVD. No anterior cervical lymphadenopathy.

Heart: RRR no murmurs/rubs/gallops. Clear S1/S2. Pulses 2+ throughout. Cap refill <2 secs.

Lungs: Clear to auscultation bilaterally. No wheezes, rubs, or rhonchi.

Abdomen: Soft non-tender. No hepatosplenomegally. +BSs. No ttp. No masses felt. Neg Murphy's sign. No rebound tenderness.

Lower extremities: No swelling, tenderness, or erythema. Negative Homan's sign. Symmetric lower extremities.

Differential Diagnosis: In order of likelihood (with 1 being the most likely), list up to 5 potential or possible diagnoses for this patient's presentation (in many cases, fewer than 5 diagnoses are likely)	Diagnostic Work-up: List immediate plans (up to 5) for further diagnostic work-up
1. Myocardial infarction	1. ECG
2. Gastroesophageal reflux disease (GERD)	2. Cardiac enzymes (Troponin, CK-MB, CK)
3. Pulmonary embolism	3. CBC with differential
4. Dissection of the large vessels	4. CXR (PA/Lat)
5. Pneumonia	5. CT angiogram, chest

12　Chronic Cough

1. Opening Scenario

Thom Nordstrom, a 65-year-old male, presents to the clinic with complaints of cough for the last 4 months.

2. Vital Signs

BP:	136/78 mmHg
Temp:	98.6° F (37.0° C)
HR:	75/minute, regular
RR:	16/minute
Pulse oximetry:	98% on room air

3. Examinee Tasks

1. Obtain a focused history.

2. Perform a relevant physical examination. (Do not perform breast, pelvic/genital, or rectal examination.)

3. Discuss your initial diagnostic impression and your work-up plan.

4. After leaving the room, complete your patient note on the given form.

Are the Vital Signs Stable?

Subjective

Knock; enter. Introduce yourself, and place the first signpost.

"Hello, Mr. Nordstrom, I'm Dr. Ashton. I understand you've been having a cough. Please tell me more about this."

"Hello Dr. Ashton. My **cough** has been around a long time. It's not a big deal or anything, but it sure is **annoying** me. Is there anything you can do?"

"Well, let me ask a few questions and I hope to be able to get to the bottom of it. When did the cough start?"

"About **4 months ago** or so. I **don't know what brought it on** but it's been since then. It started off as sort of just **clearing my throat**, you know? Then I think it got irritated and then increased. I didn't think it was anything at first. Like, it'd go away, you know, but it just keeps hanging on and on."

"That must be hard to deal with. Would you say this is a dry cough or are you bringing anything up with it?"

"No, it's a **dry cough**. About a month ago I **had a cold** and I coughed some and it brought some mucous up, but then that went away and the cough was still there, just like always."

"Have you tried anything for it? That is, have you taken any medications?"

"Yeah, I took **Sudafed** , I took a lot of **lozenges**—you know, the menthol kind? When I had a sore throat I also gargled a lot. The lozenges helped a little, but there's so many of those I can take."

"I can imagine. Those lozenges can be strong. Have you taken any antihistamines, like Benedryl?"

"Um, **no**, I can't say I have."

"When would you say the cough is worse? At night or in the daytime?"

"I'd say all day it's about the same."

"Does it ever keep you up at night?"

"Now that you mention it, it doesn't keep me up, but it makes **it kind of harder to go to sleep**. I'm trying to clear my throat at night and stuff."

"Ok. Have you seen any other doctor for this? Or been treated in the past for this type of thing?"

"**No**, I see my regular doctor about once a month for other issues. I told her about the cough, but it seems like there's always something else going on at the time of the appointment. We never really get down to talking about just the cough."

"Sometimes it can be hard to fit everything in, can't it? Well, please briefly tell me some of the other issues you're having."

"Oh, well, we talk about things like my **high cholesterol**, which has come down recently, and **high blood pressure,** I also treat that with medicine. I had some **chest pain** a couple of months ago and stayed in the emergency room overnight and she ran some tests on me after that happened. She also adjusts my other medicines."

"Ok. What medicines are those?"

"I take **lovastatin**, a cholesterol drug, **benazepril,** and another called **hydrochlorothiazide** for blood pressure. I have some inhaler medicine called **Advair** for my lungs, and I take **aspirin** once a day. I also take one called **prazosin** for my prostate."

"Ok. Are any of those new or have you started them in the past 4 months, since this cough started?"

"Oh, I don't think so. I've been on most of them for a while now, at least a year. My doctor starts them and I change dosages maybe a little and get blood taken but I've been on them for quite some time. I take that back...the **prazosin** has been in the **last 3 months**. That's it."

Asking for history of common over-the-counter medicines can sometimes jar the patient's memory about previous medications.

Never criticize a colleague to a patient if they complain about poor service.

"Ok. Just from you telling me those medicines, it seems like you have a few different types of illnesses. Can you tell me what health problems you have?"

"Sure, I've got high **blood pressure** and a **big prostate**. I've also got **high cholesterol** and something my doctor calls **COPD** from smoking."

"Ok. Besides this cough, have you had any other health problems you'd like to mention today?"

"**No**, that's it, really. My wife is on me more and more about my health. I like my doctor, too, so I try to work with her on this stuff. My daughter is a nurse and she pushes me all the time to come see you guys."

"Well, that sounds like a good thing, your family being so concerned. You said earlier you had some chest pain and stayed the night in the emergency room. Did the doctors tell you that you had any problems with your heart or lungs?"

"**No**, it was a false alarm. They said they didn't know what it was but that it wasn't anything to worry about. I think someone said it was my bones in my chest. I did a lot of tests for that—a treadmill run and a bunch of those ECGs. But eventually, it wasn't a big deal."

"Ok. How about any problems eating or with heartburn after you eat?"

"Well, I do get some **heartburn** like everyone else after I eat something **spicy**. My wife knows what I can't eat so she doesn't cook it. I've had heartburn since I was about 40 years old. I stay away from **tomatoes** and **coffee**. Sometimes I chew those calcium pills at night. I guess that chest pain could have been that but they didn't think so at the time."

"Ok. How many nights a week would you say you get the heartburn?"

"Oh, about **one or two** times. I usually take at least a few of those chewable tablets after dinner because if I don't it tends to come on after I lay down. Sometimes I don't have it at all though."

"Does the cough get worse when you have the heartburn?"

"Oh, I don't know. **Maybe**, I never thought about it."

"Ok. Have you taken any medicines for the heartburn other than the chewable tablets?"

"Well, **no**. I tried some of that other stuff, it was a little red pill, about a year ago but stopped. It didn't do much, and my doctor at the time said it might cause some problems with my other medicines. I didn't think it helped much and I just stopped eating that food that caused it. That was easier."

"Ok. Have you had a problem swallowing lately? That is, does it feel like food ever becomes stuck in your throat?"

"**No**, not that."

"You mentioned you have COPD from smoking; do you still smoke?"

"Yeah, doc. I smoke about **half a pack per day** still. My wife's especially on me about that. I was smoking about one to two packs per day for the last 30 years though, so I think I'm doing better. My doctor says that's what caused my breathing problems."

Patients often don't remember the correct past diagnosis from an incident but know fragments of related information.

With vague history, never assume what medication the patient has taken, even though they might describe it.

No matter what etiology of cough, smoking significantly worsens symptoms.

"Well, it probably has something to do with it. Do you want to completely quit?"

"**No**, not really. It's the last vice I have."

"Ok. Have you had any surgeries in your life?"

"Yeah, I had my appendix out 6 years ago. I also had a hernia fixed about a year later. Those are the only times I've had surgery."

"Ok. Do you drink alcohol?"

"I have **one beer** with dinner or after dinner when I watch TV. I don't drink any more than that."

"Ok. Has any one in your family had anything like this cough at all?"

"**No**, no one I know of. My father's dead from a **heart attack** when he was 72 years old. My **mother** died about 2 years ago from a **car accident**. She stayed 2 weeks in the ICU before she passed. She was 88 years old though. Everyone else is pretty healthy."

"That sounds like it must have been hard on everyone."

"Yeah, you know. It was hard on us all. My sister really had a tough time. Anyway, I'd rather go like my dad, frankly."

"Do you ever get depressed about your mom passing or anything else?"

"Nah, I'm sort of happy by nature. You know, when it's your time, it's your time. I was sad when she died but I've been fine for a long time now."

Signpost for the Physical Exam

"Ok. I'd like to do a physical exam now, if you don't mind. Just let me wash my hands. It looks like your **vital signs are normal.** First, let me take a look at your mouth and throat…"

Objective

Points for Every Exam:

- Wash hands.
- Comment on vital signs, even if normal.
- Tell the patient where you are going to examine and disrobe.
- Do not repeat painful maneuvers.

Physical Exam:

Perform a focused physical, by system, from the head down.

System	Exam elements	Findings in this patient
HEENT	Ears: Use the otoscope without the insuflator bulb to check for gross TM abnormalities. Nose: Assess the nasal mucosa and visible turbinates for abnormalities or hyperemia.Throat: Use the otoscope light to examine the mouth, teeth, and visible pharynx. Consider a tongue depressor if the posterior wall is not clearly visible.	Ears: TMs appear pearly gray bilaterally. Nose: pink and normal mucosa and turbinates. Throat: no erythema, tonsilor hypertrophy, or tonsilor exudates.
Lung	Listen to 6 different areas of the posterior lung fields. Comment aloud on rales, rhonchi, or wheezes.	Clear to auscultation bilaterally. No rales, rhonchi, or wheezes.

Heart	Listen to four different areas on the anterior chest.	Regular, rate, and rhythm. No murmurs, rubs, or clicks heard.
Abdomen	Listen for bowel sounds and bruit's. Palpate all 4 quadrants with the epigastrum the last area to concentrate on. Be aware of any masses that may be felt. Check Murphy's sign.	Bowel sounds normal. No hepatomegally. No peritoneal signs. The patient reports mild discomfort with direct pressure to the epigastrum. Negative Murphy's sign.

Continue to gather information as you do the physical exam. Comment aloud on any real or simulated abnormalities.

Example: *"Does it hurt when I push in here?*[when applying direct pressure to the epigastrum]*"*

Example: *"Have you had the sniffles lately?"*

End of Case

End by explaining you have several ideas of what could be wrong and could cause these symptoms. Tell the patient the first two diagnoses on your differential list and the major tests you'd now like to perform.

Example: *"Mr. Nordstrom, after listening to your symptoms and performing that physical exam, I think there are several factors that could be causing your cough. First, you might be having more severe gastric reflux, or heartburn, than we thought. With the frequency of your symptoms, I wouldn't be surprised if you were having some reflux of the stomach contents into your esophagus, or the tube connecting your mouth to your stomach. That reflux can sometimes irritate your throat and cause you to cough. For this possibility, I think it would be useful to measure the amount of acid you have in your esophagus with what's called a pH probe. The probe would be placed into your esophagus for 24 hours and measure how much acid there is; that will tell us how severe your reflux is. The probe is very small and shouldn't even be noticed much at all. Another possibility is that the medicine your on, the benazepril, is causing a side effect. That medicine is well-known for being associated with a cough and thus may just be the culprit for this problem. Yet another possibility is that your COPD, or the disease process that is going on in your lungs from the smoking, is causing your cough. Because you still smoke, it may be worsened by this and lead to your symptoms. Very rarely, this type of thing could be caused by a special type of cancer that occurs in the area of your lower throat. It's not very likely, but I'd like to do a test to evaluate for this rarity. It's called a laryngoscopy and involves numbing you up and then basically using a camera on the end of a long probe to actually look at your nose and throat. It's an in-office procedure and not anything you need to be sedated for. I'd like to step out now and arrange some of these tests with my nurse if you don't have any questions for me at this point.*

Is there any other aspect of your health care we haven't already discussed? Ok then, thank you."

PATIENT NOTE

History: Include significant positives and negatives from history of present illness, past medical history, review of system(s), social history, and family history.

HPI: 65 y/o male c/o chronic cough x 4 months. Denies URI symptoms or new medications on onset. Described as dry cough that is constant throughout the day; does affect going to sleep at night. Pt admitted to URI symptoms approximately 1 month ago that turned the cough to productive of clear mucous which has ceased since then. Accompanying symptoms include heartburn approx 1-2 nights per week requiring frequent calcium chewables. History of heavy smoking with current habit ½ ppd with concurrent COPD. Patient has taken ARB for approximately 1 year but reports possible increase in dosage over the time-course of this illness.

PMH: Hypertension, BPH, hypercholesterolemia, COPD. One episode chest pain with evaluation reported as noncardiac.

PSH: Appendectomy, hernia repair.

Tobacco: 1/2 pack per day. 40 pack-years.

Alcohol use: One drink per day.

Meds: Hydrochlorothiazide, benazepril, lovastatin, Advair, prazosin, calcium antacid tablets, and aspirin.

Physical Examination: Indicate only pertinent positive and negative findings related to the patient's chief complaint.

VS Stable.

HEENT: Ears: TMs pearly gray. Nose: Normal pink mucosa. Throat: Normal oral mucosa, no pharyngeal erythema, no tonsilor hypertrophy, no tonsilor exudates.

Lung: Clear to auscultation. No rhonchi, rales, or wheezes.

Heart: Regular, rate, and rhythm.

Abdomen: Soft, nontender. +Bowel sounds. No hepatomegally. No masses. Mild ttp of the epigastric region.

Differential Diagnosis: In order of likelihood (with 1 being the most likely), list up to 5 potential or possible diagnoses for this patient's presentation (in many cases, fewer than 5 diagnoses are likely)	Diagnostic Work-up: List immediate plans (up to 5) for further diagnostic work-up.
1. Gastroesophageal reflux disease (GERD)	1. Laryngoscopy
2. Medication effect from ACE-I medication	2. 24-hour esophageal pH probe
3. Chronic Obstructive Pulmonary Disease (COPD)	3.
4. Postinfectious cough	4.
5. Laryngeal cancer	5.

13 Shortness of Breath

1. Opening Scenario

Albert Baxter, a 65-year-old male, presents to the emergency department with increasing shortness of breath.

2. Vital Signs

BP:	146/92 mmHg
Temp:	98.9° F (37.2° C)
HR:	70/minute, regular
RR:	20/minute
Pulse oximetry:	96% on room air

3. Examinee Tasks

1. Obtain a focused history.

2. Perform a relevant physical examination. (Do not perform breast, pelvic/genital, or rectal examination.)

3. Discuss your initial diagnostic impression and your work-up plan.

4. After leaving the room, complete your patient note on the given form.

Are the Vital Signs Stable?

Subjective

Knock; enter. Introduce yourself and place the first signpost.

"Hi Mr. Baxter, I'm Dr. Stromly. I understand you've had some shortness of breath recently. Please tell me more about it."

"Hi doc. Yeah, I've had a **hard time breathing** lately. It's that I feel like I'm **not getting enough air**. I just can't seem to breathe deep enough to get enough air, and that gives me a very uncomfortable feeling. I feel like I'm panting like crazy."

"I can imagine that it does. How long have you felt like this?"

"It's been **increasing for the last week**. But it's been the **last few days** it's been the worst. You know, it's **worse at night**, though. I get more **tired** during the day, too. It's like I'm just **exhausted a little**

while after I wake up. It's harder and harder to even function outside a lounge chair, doc."

"Has this ever happened to you before or is this the first time?"

"Yeah, well, I've been tired before, sure, but **not like this**. I've felt like lying around all day and then haven't been able to sleep at night because I have trouble breathing."

"Ok. Have you had trouble breathing when you exert yourself a little during the day, too, or is it mainly when you lay down?"

"Yeah, I'd say when I **exert myself**. I went to the post office today and went to mail a heavy box and had to stop and catch my breath when I took it to the counter. I mean, look at me; I've never had to do that. Besides that, it's mainly when I lay down at night. It's not immediately, but it **takes a while** then it's worse."

"That's unusual, huh? Have you had any chest pain with this?"

"Well, I've been trying to think of that since the nurse asked me the same question. I'd say **'yes'** for the past **few days**. I couldn't actually say pain as much as **pressure** in my chest, right about here [placing his right hand on his **left chest wall**]. It feels **heavy**, especially when I breathe in, you know. That's only there when I move around a lot, though. It's **not like my usual heartburn**, but more of a heavy-type feeling."

"Ok. How long would you say that's been going on?"

"Well, since the shortness of breath got real bad. That's since Friday, so **2 days now**. It's not very bad, but it's there."

"Does that feeling radiate to your arms or up to your neck?"

"**No**, it just stays there."

"You said that's worse with exertion, as well, so on a scale of 0 to 10, 10 being the worst pain imaginable, where would you put that feeling?"

"Oh, well, I would only say about a **3 or 4**. Not that bad."

"Does anything make it better?"

"Well, it's not there when I'm **resting**. That's about it."

"Ok. How about any other symptoms, such as wheezing when you breathe? That is, do you ever notice a high-pitched sound when you breathe, sort of a whistle that is commonly present when you exhale?"

"**Yeah**, I do wheeze, actually. Sometimes I get up at night with that. I **sleep with three pillows behind my head**, because I have heartburn, you know, and if I roll off them in the middle of the night, I get up and notice that. That just started over the last week, though, now that you mention it."

"Do you mean the wheezing?"

"Yeah, and the getting up in the middle of the night if I roll off the pillows. That's because of the shortness of breath."

"Have you ever had trouble breathing before?"

"I used to **smoke cigarettes** and my doctor said I had something called **COPD**. He said if I don't quit I'd get lung cancer or emphysema. So I quit. That was about **2 years ago,** but I had smoked for **30 years** before

Delayed orthopnea is a hallmark of paroxysmal nocturnal dyspnea (PND) caused by CHF.

Thoroughly explain all medical terms, especially specific symptoms.

that. That was at a **pack and a half to two packs a day**. So then I just had enough and quit, but I already did some damage, he said, and I could expect some lung problems."

"Well, congratulations on quitting smoking. The key is keeping off the cigarettes. Have you had any other symptoms besides the ones we've already talked about?"

"I don't think so. Oh, I've also had a **cough** with all this, if that means anything. I think I have a cold, honestly, but I'm losing sleep because of the thing."

"Is that more at night or during the day?"

"Oh, at **night** is when I notice it."

"Have you had any fever, or do you bring up anything with that cough?"

"**No**, it's just a dry-type cough. **No fever,** although I haven't taken my temperature either."

"How about any other problems with things like puffiness of your hands and feet or turning blue?"

"I've been feeling like **my hands have been puffy** for a while. And my **legs** are that way, too. I guess I haven't made much out of it though. I've never turned blue."

"How about any increase in your belly size or weight gain?"

"Well, nothing that I can blame on a disease, doc. I've **put on a few pounds** over the years but I'm the only one to blame for that."

"It's easy to let some things go sometimes. But do you think that weight has been gradual over the years or in the last few months?

"Umm, maybe more in the last few months. The thing I guess is the swelling in my legs, now that you said that. They've gotten bigger, but I just don't mind it much."

"Are you having any pain in your legs?"

"**No**, not really, no pain."

"Okay. How about any problems thinking or feeling dizzy?"

"**Nope**, not at all."

"Going back to the time you smoked and what your doctor told you when you quit, did you ever have to take a medicine for breathing problems?"

"I was on **albuterol**, the puffing medicine, for a while. I took it sometimes but really didn't feel like I needed it every day. So, I **only take it when I need it** now."

"Have you taken it lately?"

"**Yeah**, I took it **yesterday** and **the day before** but it just hasn't gotten any better. It's been a while since my last refill, though, so the medicine might not be working because it might have expired. I also don't like to take it at night because it **keeps me from sleeping**, you know."

"Yeah, I know it can have that effect. Have you taken anything else besides that inhaled medicine? Any other medications at all?"

"Oh, well, sure. I'm on a bunch of them. Let's see…I take atenolol and lisinopril for blood pressure, I take lovastatin for my cholesterol, albuterol for

Take every opportunity to congratulate the patient on quitting smoking.

It's important to ascertain if weight gain is to the result of water retention or increased obesity. Time-course may help.

lung problems, omeprazole for heartburn and reflux, and I also take my insulin for my diabetes. I also take an aspirin every day."

"Ok. Let me ask what your regimen is for taking that insulin?"

"I take **regular insulin** 15 units in the morning and 20 units at night. I also take **glargine** insulin 30 units at night. That was the last change my doctor made with me about **2 months ago**. My blood sugars seem to be high, a lot, so we changed it."

"What are some examples of your typical blood sugar readings?"

"Oh, **170, 180**. In that range."

"Ok. Have you had any problems from diabetes? Such as been admitted to the hospital or your doctor ever mentioning eye or kidney problems?"

"**No**, I've never been in the hospital for it. My doctor keeps testing me for kidney problems, he keeps taking urine when I see him, but there's no problem so far."

"Ok. So as far as health problems, I have that you have high blood pressure, high cholesterol, diabetes, reflux disease, COPD, along with these new complaints that you came in for. Are there any other medical problems I should know about?"

"Well, I think that's enough. **Nothing** else."

"Have you ever had surgery?"

"Oh, **yeah**. I've had several **hernias** in my groin. Both sides, but then the right side came loose and they had to redo it. I also **had my appendix out**. These surgeries were years ago, though."

"Ok. Are you allergic to anything?"

"I get a **rash** when I take **sulfa** drugs."

"What about drinking alcohol?"

"**No**, I don't drink anymore."

"Ok. Are there any major health problems in your family?"

"I have an **aunt with melanoma**. My mom and dad are both dead years now. My **dad** died of **lung cancer** at age **71,** and my **mom** died from **breast cancer** when she was just **62 years old**. That was a long time ago. My brothers both have **diabetes** like me. One had a **heart attack last year**, he was 62 years old, but he lived through this one."

> In patients with IDDM, two important questions to answer are: "How much insulin are you on?" and "What are your typical blood sugar readings?"

> Pertinent family history generally only includes first-degree relatives.

Signpost for the Physical Exam

"Ok. I'd like to do a physical exam now, if you don't mind. Just let me **wash my hands.** I'd first like to start by examining your neck..."

Objective

Points for Every Exam:

- Wash hands.

- Comment on vital signs, even if normal.
- Tell the patient where you are going to examine and disrobe.
- Do not repeat painful maneuvers.

Physical Exam:

Perform a focused physical, by system, from the head down.

System	Exam elements	Findings in this patient
Neck	Examine the anterior and posterior lymph node chains, commenting aloud on any abnormalities. Listen to the carotid areas for bruit's. Check the jugular venous distension and the hepatojugular reflex.	No lymphadenopathy, no carotid bruit's. Moderate JVD, positive hepatojugular reflex.
Heart	Listen to at least 4 different auscultation points on the anterior chest. Check the peripheral pulses and assess for dependent edema in lower extremities, lumbar back, and hands.	Regular rate and rhythm. Normal S1/S2. S3 is present. No rubs, no murmurs. 2+ pitting edema in lower extremities. 1+ pitting edema in hands. No edema in lumbar region. Pulses normal and symmetric throughout.
Lung	Ask the patient to take several deep breaths through an open mouth. Listen to at least 6 auscultation points on the posterior lung fields, with special attention to the bases. Comment on the presence of rales/rhonchi/rubs/wheezes. Listen for egophony.	Good breath sounds throughout both lung fields. Positive rales heard at bilateral lung bases (approx 1/3 of the distance up the posterior lung fields). No rhonchi or wheezes. No egophony.
Abdomen	Assess the size of the liver with percussion. Check for abdominal ascites with fluid wave maneuvers. Listen for bowel sounds and palpate for tenderness or masses.	No hepatosplenomegally. Negative fluid wave. Normal bowel sounds without tenderness or masses.

Continue to gather information as you do the physical exam. Comment aloud on any real or simulated abnormalities.

Example: *"Please cough for me a few times while I listen to your back."*

Example: *"Have you noticed increasing your notches on your belt recently?"*

TABLE 13.1 A Selection of Cardiac Abnormalities and the Expected Clinical Findings.

Abnormality	Primary site of murmur	Radiation	Timing	Added sounds*	Graphical Representation of the sounds
Aortic stenosis	'Aortic area' and apex	To carotid arteries	Ejection systolic	Ejection click (esp. bicuspid valve)	
Aortic regurgitation	Left sternal edge	Towards apex	Early diastolic	(Austin-Flint murmur)	
Mitral stenosis	Apex	Nil	Mid-diastolic	Opening snap	
Mitral regurgitation	Apex	Toward left axilla or base of left lung	Pansystolic	Mid-systolic click (if prolapsing)	

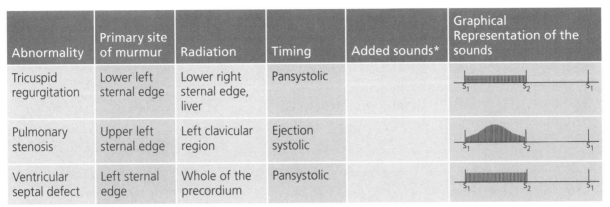

Abnormality	Primary site of murmur	Radiation	Timing	Added sounds*	Graphical Representation of the sounds
Tricuspid regurgitation	Lower left sternal edge	Lower right sternal edge, liver	Pansystolic		
Pulmonary stenosis	Upper left sternal edge	Left clavicular region	Ejection systolic		
Ventricular septal defect	Left sternal edge	Whole of the precordium	Pansystolic		

*Note that added sounds such as clicks and snaps may only be present in certain patients and should not be "expected" when examining someone with a certain abnormality.

Reprinted with permission from Thomas & Monahan. *Oxford Handbook of Clinical Examination and Practical Skills.* Oxford University Press, 2007.

End of Case

End by explaining you have several ideas of what could be wrong and could cause these symptoms. Tell the patient the first two diagnoses on your differential list and the major tests you'd now like to perform.

Example: *"Mr. Baxter, after talking with you and doing your physical exam, there are several possibilities that could be at work causing your symptoms. One possibility is that you have a disease called congestive heart failure, which is the inability of your heart to properly pump blood to the body. It happens in many people because of various reasons ranging from high blood pressure to arterial disease in the heart to even a heart attack. It's serious in that when the heart slows down and stops pumping blood effectively out of the lungs and into the body, fluid may build up in these places, causing symptoms like breathing problems or puffiness in the lower legs. This could be what's happening with you. To evaluate this, I'll need to get an X-ray of your chest and some blood work. Another possibility is that you did actually have a small heart attack. In fact, that could lead to the heart failure I just described. In people who are diabetic, the chances of actually feeling a heart attack in the typical way goes down because of problems the disease causes with nerves. Thus, you might not have even known it. For that possibility, I'd like to get an ECG, or an electrical picture of your heart, and some other blood work. There are some other possibilities, too, which I can also evaluate with the blood work and tests I'm going to get. Please allow me to step out and arrange for these tests so we can determine better what might be going on.*

Is there any other aspect of your health care we haven't already discussed? Ok then, thank you."

PATIENT NOTE

History: Include significant positives and negatives from history of present illness, past medical history, review of system(s), social history, and family history.

HPI: 65 y/o male presents to ER for increasing SOB and DOE x 2 days. Symptoms have increased for the last week but have noticably worsened over 2 days accompanied by fatigue, weakness, nocturnal wheezing, nocturnal cough, and chest "pressure". Pressure in chest described as heavy feeling beginning 2 days ago, 3-4/10 intensity, without radiation, worsened with exertion, and relieved by rest. He also admits to worsening peripheral edema but denies ascites or generalized fever. PND described with use of three pillows at night to prop head up although states he does this because of GERD symptoms.

PMH: IDDM, hypercholesterolemia, GERD, hypertension, COPD.

PSH: Hernia repair x 3–historic; appendectomy–historic.

Tobacco: Quit x 2 years, 60 pack-years.

EtOH: Denies.

Meds: Atenolol, lisinopril, atorvastatin, aspirin, omeprazole, albuterol–occasional, insulin Regular 15 u qam, 20 u qpm, Glargine 30 u qpm.

Allergies: Sulpha.

FamH: Father—deceased, lung cancer; mother—deceased, breast cancer; siblings—DM and MI x 1.

Physical Examination: Indicate only pertinent positive and negative findings related to the patient's chief complaint.

VS Stable. Elevated BP noted.

Neck: Normal appearance. No lymphadenopathy, no carotid bruit's. Moderate JVD, positive hepatojugular reflex.

Heart: Regular rate and rhythm. Normal S1/S2. Positive S3. No rubs, no murmurs. 2+ pitting edema in lower extremities. 1+ pitting edema in hands. No edema in lumbar region. Pulses normal and symmetric throughout.

Lungs: Good air movement throughout bilateral lung fields. Positive rales heard at bilateral lung bases extending cephalad approximately 1/3 the lung field. No rhonchi or wheezes. No egophony.

Abdomen: No hepatosplenomegally. Negative fluid wave. Normal bowel sounds without tenderness or masses.

Differential Diagnosis: In order of likelihood (with 1 being the most likely), list up to 5 potential or possible diagnoses for this patient's presentation (in many cases, fewer than 5 diagnoses are likely)	Diagnostic Work-up: List immediate plans (up to 5) for further diagnostic work-up
1. Congestive heart failure exacerbation	1. Chest X-ray
2. Myocardial infarction	2. CBC with differential, electrolytes, renal function, glucose
3. COPD exacerbation	3. Cardiac enzymes (Troponin, CK-MB, CPK)
4. Pneumonia	4. ECG
5. Pulmonary emobolism	5. B-type naturetic peptide (BNP)

---

1. Opening Scenario

Allan Cuchet, a 57-year-old male, comes to the clinic complaining of unintentional weight loss and fatigue.

2. Vital Signs

BP:	132/86 mmHg
Temp:	98.7° F (37.1° C)
HR:	76/minute, regular
RR:	16/minute
Weight:	277 lbs (126 kg)
Height:	6′2″ (188 cm)
BMI:	35.6 kg/m²

3. Examinee Tasks

1. Obtain a focused history.

2. Perform a relevant physical examination. (Do not perform breast, pelvic/genital, or rectal examination.)

3. Discuss your initial diagnostic impression and your work-up plan.

4. After leaving the room, complete your patient note on the given form.

Are the Vital Signs Stable?

Subjective

Knock; enter. Introduce yourself, and place the first signpost.

"Hi, Mr Cuchet, I'm Dr. Dietz. I understand you've had some unusual symptoms of weight loss and feeling tired lately. Please tell me more about it."

"Hey, yeah, honestly doc, I've been **feeling tired** as heck lately, and I don't know why. I'm a foreman down at Click's construction and have worked there for 21 years. Lately, I can't seem to pull myself out of a rut all day. I'm just so tired. My wife says I've been sulking around the house for weeks,

> If the patient doesn't volunteer it, an occupational history is very important in the complaint of fatigue.

but honestly, it's just because I don't have the energy at night anymore, either."

"Really? Has this started recently or been going on a long time?"

"Oh it's been for **about a month** now, I s'pose, although it's been building now for some time."

"Have you changed your sleeping habits or what you do at home at night?"

"**Nope**, like clockwork, I read in bed until about 10:30 then fall asleep… although recently it's been sooner…maybe 10. I get up at 6:15 every morning; that hasn't changed in 20 years."

"Have you ever lost consciousness unexpectedly during the day?"

"**No**, I'm just sleepy all the time."

"How much caffeine do you drink?"

"Well, I have about **half a pot of coffee** in the morning, that's it."

"Do you smoke?"

"I **haven't smoked in the last 10 years**, although before that I smoked **a pack a day for 12 years**. That coffee habit hasn't changed though, and I'm getting the **same amount of sleep** I've always gotten."

"I noticed you also said you'd been losing weight, too? How much have you lost?"

"Yeah, I wouldn't have noticed except my belt has gotten much looser in the last few weeks. **I went down two belt notches,** and my wife keeps saying there's something wrong because I still eat a lot. I **haven't tried** to lose weight, it's just sort of happening. I haven't actually stepped on a scale in years though—never needed to."

"Do you exercise regularly?"

"I **don't go to the gym** if that's what you're asking. I've always gotten enough exercise at work. My other doctor's always on me about that, too."

"Well, I don' want to sound like I'm admonishing you. Have there been any other symptoms at all?"

"Well, it also seems like **I'm always thirsty** lately. I don't mean alcohol; I just mean stuff like water and soda. Seems like I'm **peeing** like a too, pardon the expression."

"Really? How about burning when you urinate? Or problems starting a urine stream?"

"No problems actually peeing—just happens so often."

"You mentioned thirst. Has there been a change recently?"

"Yeah, I work outside most of the day, and it's hot. But this **drinking much more than usual** seems strange, you know? Not a big deal. It's the feeling of being tired that's the real problem."

"Ok. How about other things, like blurring of your vision?"

"**No**, I wear these glasses, but I **haven't noticed** a problem with the prescription lately."

"Have you had any headaches or a stiff neck recently?"

> A detailed sleep history should be obtained in anyone with chronic fatigue.

> Common stimulants to ask about are caffeine and nicotine.

"Not anything unusual, from time to time I get headaches and stiff muscles but no increase in that. Sometimes I **get winded climbing stairs** at work, but as you can see, I'm a big guy."

"How about chest pain or feeling like your heart is racing? Any problems like this in your family?"

"**Nope**, haven't had any problems with the ticker. My **dad died of a heart attack** 2 years ago; he was **77 years old**, and my mom's still around."

"How about nausea or problems with having a bowel movement?"

"No, I go once in the morning **everyday,** and like I said, I **eat like crazy lately**."

"Have you noticed any problems with sensation in your hands or moving your arms or legs?"

"Oh **no**, I'm a foreman. I have to be able to move around, no problems."

"Alright. Tell me, have you ever seen the doctor for anything serious in your life? Especially anything you've spent the night in the hospital for?"

"Yeah, back about 6 or 7 years ago, I got my hand caught in a chain mixer. It tore a big hole in my arm and broke it up pretty good. They fixed that with **three surgeries,** but it works good now. My other doctor also told me I have high blood pressure, and he's got me on these pills. They made me pee like crazy in the beginning but that's stopped now. Started them about 5 years ago, **blood pressure has been fine** on every visit since. I also take a new one for high cholesterol. I think its called lovastatin; I just started that 6 months ago and haven't had any problems."

> If a major disease such as diabetes, hypertension, or heart disease is high on your differential, then assess for risk factors of the disease.

"Let's go back to your family; did anyone have any major diseases like diabetes or cancer?"

"Well, my **dad did have diabetes** when I was a kid. He was also a big man, **315 pounds** when he died of that heart attack. And my brother has **lung cancer** but was treated. My mom's healthy as an ox, though."

"Ok. Just a few more questions, do you drink alcohol or have you in the past?"

"I have a **beer with dinner** at night, but I'm too old to do much more drinking. As a younger man, but those days are far behind me."

"How about allergies? Especially to medication?"

"**Nope**, nothing I know of."

"What medications did you say you were on?"

"Yeah, its **hydrochlorothiazide**. I take 25 milligrams a day. I remember because it has that long name. Then that lovastatin. I'm not on anything else except for the occasional **Tylenol**."

Signpost for the Physical Exam

"Ok. I'd like to do a physical exam now, if you don't mind. Just let me wash my hands. It looks like your **vital signs are normal,** so please let me first look at your eyes…"

Objective

Points for Every Exam:

- Wash hands.
- Comment on vital signs, even if normal.
- Tell the patient where you are going to examine and disrobe.
- Do not repeat painful maneuvers.

Physical Exam:

Perform a focused physical, by system, from the head down.

System	Exam elements	Findings in this patient
Eyes	Examine the pupils, external eye, and perform a retinal exam.	PERRLA, normal external ocular eye movements. Retina show normal vascular and optic disc appearance.
Neurologic	Assess cranial nerves, symmetry of at least 2 different deep tendon reflexes, motor strength, tactile sensation on the hand/fingers and feet/toes. Perform monofilament testing on the feet and two-point discrimination and proprioception on the toes. Test vibration testing on hands/feet.	Normal neurologic exam, including cranial nerves, tactile sensation, proprioception, and two-point discrimination. Monofilament normal. Motor strength 5/5, symmetric. DTRs symmetric.
Respiratory	Listen to 6 auscultation points on the posterior lung fields. Note any abnormalities aloud.	Clear to auscultation. No wheezes, rales, or rhonchi.
Cardiac	Listen to 4 auscultation points, palpate radial pulses, check capillary refill.	Regular rate and rhythm. Normal radial pulses. Capillary refill <2 sec.
Abdomen	Listen for bowel sounds and bruit's, and attempt to illicit tenderness to palpation. Percuss the approximate liver size.	Obese abdomen. Liver size unable to determine. No ascites.
Skin	Check the feet for ulcerations or wounds.	Normal appearance

Continue to gather information as you do the physical exam. Ask about pertinent aspects of each system as you perform the exams. Comment aloud on any real or simulated abnormalities.

Example: *"How long have you had vision problems? [as you exam external eyes]."*

Example: *"Have you stubbed your toe recently?"*

End of Case

End by explaining you have several ideas of what could be wrong and could cause these symptoms. Tell the patient the first two diagnoses on your differential list and the major tests you'd now like to perform.

Example: *"Mr. Cuchet, your symptoms make me think of several different diseases that may be going on in your body. Specifically, diabetes and low thyroid gland function could be present as well as a few other things. We can test for the cause, and I'd like to schedule you for those tests today. We'll have to have you come back for the actual tests, however, because it will take an overnight fast from eating for a specific blood test I'd like to run called a blood glucose level. At the same time, I will obtain other blood tests to check for those other diseases I* *mentioned. While here in the clinic today, however, I'd like to take a sample of blood from your finger to just make sure your blood glucose isn't too high. I will have my nurse come in to get that quick sample of blood and to set up a time for the tests. I would also like you to schedule an appointment for a day or two after the blood is taken to discuss your results. Please make that at your convenience.*

Is there any other aspect of your health care we haven't already discussed? Ok then, thank you."

PATIENT NOTE

History: Include significant positives and negatives from history of present illness, past medical history, review of system(s), social history, and family history.

HPI: 57 y/o male with fatigue and weight loss. The fatigue started about 1 month ago with gradual onset and is not accompanied by change in sleep habits or caffeine/stimulant intake. He has not had LOC during daily activities and does not believe it's caused by inadequate sleep. He also notes recent unintentional weight loss although isn't able to state how much. He states he has increased thirst and urination although denies other urinary symptoms. No change in eating habits although question of polyphagia.

ROS: No vision changes, wears glasses. No change in sensation or loss of motor control. No chest pain or palpitations. No change in bowel habits.

Meds: Hydrochlorothiazide and lovastatin. No change in dosage. Occasional Tylenol.

PMH: Hypertension—treated. Hypercholesterolemia—treated.

PSH: Arm fracture requiring ORIF 6–7 years ago.

Smoking: Quit x 10 years. 12 pack-years.

Alcohol use: Approximately 1 drink per day.

Allergies: NKA.

FamH: Father—deceased of MI, age 77 years, also had DM and obesity; brother—lung cancer.

Physical Examination: Indicate only pertinent positive and negative findings related to the patient's chief complaint.

VS Stable, normal.

Gen: Overweight.

HEENT: Eyes PERLA, retinal vasculature and optic disc normal bilaterally. Thyroid not enlarged, nontender.

Neuro: Strength 5/5 throughout, Reflexes 2+ biceps and quads. Sensation: tactile sense normal bilateral hands. Feet show two point discrimination normal. Normal sharp/dull testing. Vibration sense normal. Monofilament normal bilaterally on feet.

Heart: RRR no murmurs, rubs, gallops. Pulse's normal-radial and dorsalis pedis.

Abdomen: Obese. Soft, nontender. Normal bowel sounds. No abdominal bruit's. No masses or ttp.

Extremities: No pitting edema, no skin changes.

Differential Diagnosis: In order of likelihood (with 1 being the most likely), list up to 5 potential or possible diagnoses for this patient's presentation (in many cases, fewer than 5 diagnoses are likely)	Diagnostic Work-up: List immediate plans (up to 5) for further diagnostic work-up
1. Diabetes Mellitis	1. Finger-stick glucose level
2. Hyperthyroid state	2. TSH, Free T4
3. Diabetes Insipidus	3. CBC with differential
4. Cushing's syndrome	4. Complete metabolic profile
5. Occult malignancy	5. Fasting glucose level

15   Respiratory Symptoms

1. Opening Scenario

Andre McCormitt, a 59-year-old male, presents with complaints of chest congestion and cough.

2. Vital Signs

BP:	139/78 mmHg
Temp:	101.1° F (38.4° C)
HR:	66/minute, regular
RR:	16/minute
Pulse oximetry:	96% on room air

3. Examinee Tasks

1. Obtain a focused history.

2. Perform a relevant physical examination. (Do not perform breast, pelvic/genital, or rectal examination.)

3. Discuss your initial diagnostic impression and your work-up plan.

4. After leaving the room, complete your patient note on the given form.

Are the Vital Signs Stable?

Subjective

Knock; enter. Introduce yourself, and place the first signpost.

"Hello, Mr. McCormitt, I'm Dr. Lewis. I understand you've been having a cough and chest congestion lately. Please tell me more about these symptoms?"

"Yes doctor. I've been feeling just terrible. My chest's been **congested,** and I've had a **cold** for about **2 weeks**. I'm a **store owner,** and lately it's just been hard to get up in the morning and run things; I feel so **tired,** and run down, and icky. At night I **barely sleep** because I'm so **hot**. I'm also **coughing like crazy,** which keeps my wife up. Look, I'm just trying to find something else that can get me through this crud. What I have just isn't working."

"I'm sorry to hear that. How long have you had these symptoms?"

"Well, it's been about **2 weeks** since it started. My daughter, visiting from North Carolina, brought the grandkids over, and they'd recently had this cold, you know. Guess I got it from them."

"Possibly. You said you'd had chest congestion, is there any pain with that?"

"**No**, my chest just **feels heavy**, ya know? It just feels like I have a bunch of gunk in there, and it's even kind of **hard to breathe when I lie down** sometimes."

"Ok. Is it every time you lie down, or just sometimes that you have trouble breathing?"

Characterize any shortness of breath, especially when lying down. Think PND.

"Well, it's not really trouble breathing, just more of that **heavy feeling** again. It's right when I lie down but **goes away after a few minutes**. It's not like I'm gasping for air or anything."

"Ok. Tell me about that cough. Are you bringing any sputum up with that?"

"Yeah, a lot. I feel like I'm hacking up a lung most of the time. It's pretty **bad-tasting**, too."

"Is there any blood in the sputum?"

"No, not usually. I **did have some** the other day now that you mention it, but it went away. Does that mean it might be, like, lung cancer?"

Address patient concerns such as cancer and questions of life-threatening illness immediately in the conversation.

"No, it doesn't necessarily mean anything like cancer. Blood in sputum, by itself, is just another sign I want to know about because it may mean a lot of things. Cancer is one disease that may cause blood in the sputum, but that remains fairly rare compared to the other reasons. Simple cough is the most common reason causing this, and the blood often comes from the back of the throat. How much blood was there?"

"Not much, I just noticed it **stained a little pink** after a hard **coughing spell**. I've been checking since then and there's been nothing."

"What color is the sputum you're bringing up?"

"It started out white, now it's mostly a **yellow or greenish**. When I'm really coughing hard there might even be some brown."

"Ok. How about other symptoms like fever?"

"**Yeah**, I've been hot lately. At night is when I get most hot. Sometimes I **sweat** a lot. I haven't taken my temperature, but it seems high. I sometimes take some **Tylenol,** which helps, I suppose."

"Do you have chills as well or just feel hot? How about body aches?"

"**Yeah**, like I said, it's hard to get up to run my store. My whole **body just aches**, especially my **joints**. You know that feeling when you get sick? I haven't had any chills."

Don't hesitate to clarify previously mentioned illness characteristics.

"Alright. We've covered your chest congestion, cough, body aches, and subjective fever; are there any other symptoms you can tell me about? Any headache or sinus pressure?"

"No, I don't really get headaches. I had a really **stuffy nose** at the beginning of this cold but it went away."

"How about any nausea or vomiting? Is your appetite still there?"

"**No** nausea or vomiting. I still eat a lot. My wife sees to that. They say 'feed a cold, starve a fever,' don't they? That's my philosophy."

"Ok. Any diarrhea or abdominal pain?"

"**Nope**, both are normal."

"We covered your symptoms of chest congestion, but have you had any short-ness of breath, even while doing your daily activities?"

"**No**, I've been fine. I usually walk at night with my wife for exercise. I haven't lately but **no shortness of breath**."

"You said you took Tylenol. Have you taken any other medications for this or are you on any other medications for anything?"

"I've taken **Tylenol** a few times. My wife gave me some **ibuprofen**, too. I've only taken either about four times in the last few weeks. They help a little, I guess. Then I'm also on **hydrocholorthiazide** and another one called **atenolol** for my blood pressure. My other doctor also has me on **lovastatin** for my cholesterol. I've been on those for a **few years** though."

"Ok. Do you smoke? Or have you used tobacco in the past?"

"I smoke about **half a pack per day**. I've done that for about **30 years**. I smoke the light cigarettes, though, the menthol kind."

"Half a pack per day, huh? Ok. Actually it really doesn't matter to your body if the cigarette is light or not; all cigarettes are bad for you. We can talk more about that later if you'd like. I'd like to help you quit smoking if you would like to attempt it. Is that something you might be interested in?"

"Um, well…not really doc. I've done it for a heck of a long time, and I'll probably just keep on doing it. That's alright, but I'd rather just keep going."

"Alright. Well, if you'd like to attempt to quit, know that I'll be here to help.

How about drinking alcohol?"

"I **don't drink** anymore. Quit, maybe, 10 years ago. Doesn't interest me."

"How about any other illnesses you've seen the doctor for? Have you ever spent the night in the hospital?"

"Like I mentioned, I'm on those medicines from my regular doctor. Otherwise, I had a **hernia** operation a year ago. Down here in my groin [pointing to the left inguinal area]. Didn't spend the night, though. I also had a **colonoscopy** because my **brother had colon cancer** last year. Nothing else, though."

"Ok. Did the colonoscopy show anything?"

"**No,** it was clear."

"Has your regular doctor ever mentioned to you a long-term illness called 'COPD' or had breathing tests done? These would be tests where you are asked to breath forcefully into a machine that then collects data?"

"No, I haven't had any of that stuff done. Never heard of COPD, either."

"How about the word 'emphysema?'"

"Well, I've heard of that, but my doctor hasn't ever said I have it."

"Ok. How about other surgeries?"

"I broke my arm about 10 years ago, and they went and reset it. It was ok. Actually, I did stay overnight for that one. Long time ago, though."

> If the patient mentions a known myth about important health care, address it. If smoking is brought up, offer to address this concern at a later point. However, don't be distracted from the main illness in the interview.

"Ok. Have you ever had a pneumonia vaccine? It would have been a shot your doctor told you about?"

"No, is there one? I never knew."

"Yes, there is. It's not quite recommended for your age group, however. That may be why your regular doctor hasn't brought it up. Other than that colon cancer in your brother, have there been any other major diseases in your family?"

*"Jerry had that cancer. My father passed away of a **heart attack** at age 79. My mom died in a car wreck about 5 years ago now. She was 83 years old. No other cancers or problems."*

Signpost for the Physical Exam

*"Ok. I'd like to do a physical exam now, if you don't mind. Just let me wash my hands. It looks by your **vital signs** you have a **fever.** I'd like to ask you to remove your shirt so I may listen to your back and chest…"*

Objective

Points for Every Exam:

- Wash hands.
- Comment on vital signs, even if normal.
- Tell the patient where you are going to examine and disrobe.
- Do not repeat painful maneuvers.

Physical Exam:

Perform a focused physical, by system, from the head down.

System	Exam elements	Findings in this patient
HEENT	Ears: Examine the ears with an insufflator bulb, bilaterally. Eyes: Examine the conjunctivae and the pupils with a bright penlight or otoscope light. A retinal exam is not needed. Ask the patient to look toward the ceiling and open his mouth for examination of the oral cavity and visible pharynx. Use a tongue depressor and examine the teeth and gums briefly, followed by the posterior pharynx and tonsils.	Ears: TMs pearly gray bilaterally. No erythema, retractions, bulging of the TMs. Eyes: mild sclera hyperemia. PERRLA. Throat: positive postnasal drainage. Uvula midline, Mild erythema. No tonsilar swelling, no tonsilar exudates.
Lungs	Auscultate the posterior lung fields. Make sure to listen to 6 points on the posterior lung fields. If rhonchi are heard, then ask the patient to pronounce "Eee" and check for egophony.	Rhonchi are heard at each lung base. Egophony in the right lung base. No wheezing, no rales.
Heart	Auscultate at least 4 different areas of the anterior chest. Feel radial pulses, and check capillary refill.	RRR, no murmur/rub/gallop. Normal S1/S2. Pulses 2+ throughout. Cap refill <2 secs.
Abdomen	Observe the abdomen, then listen for bowel sounds or abdominal bruit's. Palpate the abdomen, asking if he is having pain in each quadrant. Check for masses (comment on lack of them), Murphy's sign, and direct/rebound tenderness over McBurney's point.	Normal BSs. Nontender and nondistended abdomen. Mildly obese.

Continue to gather information as you do the physical exam. Comment aloud on any real or simulated abnormalities.

Example: *"Does taking a deep breath make the chest heaviness worse?"*

Example: *"Please cough for me while I listen to your back."*

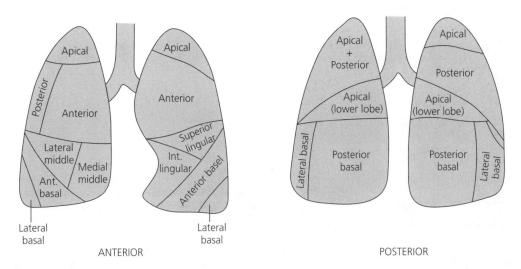

FIGURE 15.1 The respiratory segments supplied by the segmental bronchi.

Reprinted with permission from Longmore & Wilkinson. *Oxford Handbook of Clinical Medicine*, 6th ed. Oxford University Press, 2004.

End of Case

End by explaining you have several ideas of what could be wrong and could cause these symptoms. Tell the patient the first two diagnoses on your differential list and the major tests you'd now like to perform.

> **Example:** *"Mr. McCormitt, after examining you and hearing about your symptoms, I've thought of several different problems that may be going on. The most common and likely reason for all your symptoms is a viral process leading to congestion and cough from irritation of your airway. This is commonly referred to as the common cold or 'upper respiratory tract infection.' However, a cold usually gets better in a few weeks, and your fever makes me also concerned for another infection that might be caused by bacteria occurring in your lungs, such as pneumonia. Pneumonia is somewhat more serious than your common cold and may be treated with antibiotics. However, I would like to run some blood tests and have you get an X-ray of your chest to evaluate for this possibility. There are a few other possibilities that I'll also do some screening tests for in your blood, although I think these are less likely. Please allow me to step out and arrange these tests with my nurse.*
>
> *Is there any other aspect of your health care we haven't already discussed? Ok then, thank you."*

PATIENT NOTE

History: Include significant positives and negatives from history of present illness, past medical history, review of system(s), social history, and family history.

HPI: 59 y/o male c/o chest congestion and cough x 2 weeks. Symptoms started with sick contacts with similar symptoms and slowly progressed to involve "heavy

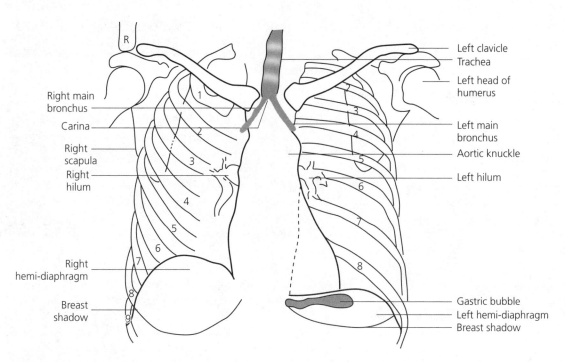

FIGURE 15.2 Structures shown on a normal chest X-ray. Numbers on left-hand side of diagram = anterior ribs and numbers on right-hand side of diagram = posterior ribs.

feeling" in chest and productive cough for yellow/green/brown sputum. Hemoptysis described only at the end of severe coughing fit. Accompanying symptoms of subjective fever and body aches with occasional return of heavy feeling in chest, although denies overt orthopnea. Denies overt SOB or DOE. He has taken PRN Tylenol and ibuprofen although minimal effect. No reported history of COPD or pulmonary function testing.

ROS: Negative for chest pain, DOE. Negative sinus pain although mild nasal symptoms at start of illness. No n/v/d.

PMH: Hypertension, hypercholesterolemia, Colonoscopy reported as negative.

PSH: Fractured arm, left inguinal hernia.

Tobacco: ½ ppd. 15 pack-years. No desire to quit.

Alcohol use: Denies.

FamH: Father—deceased, MI; mother—deceased, trauma; brother—colon cancer.

Physical Examination: Indicate only pertinent positive and negative findings related to the patient's chief complaint.

VS Stable, temperature increased.

HEENT: TMs pearly gray bilaterally, Eyes: Mild scleral hyperemia, PERRLA. Neck: No lymphadenopathy, Throat: Mild erythema, no exudates, uvula midline, no tonsilar swelling.

Lung: Positive rhonchi heard at bilateral lung bases. Egophony heard in the right lung base. No wheezing or rales.

Heart: RRR no m/r/g. Pulses 2+ throughout. Cap refill <2 secs.

Abdomen: Normal BSs, no bruit's. Nontender and nondistended abdomen. Mildly obese.

Differential Diagnosis: In order of likelihood (with 1 being the most likely), list up to 5 potential or possible diagnoses for this patient's presentation (in many cases, fewer than 5 diagnoses are likely)	Diagnostic Work-up: List immediate plans (up to 5) for further diagnostic work-up
1. Upper respiratory tract infection, viral	1. CBC with differential
2. Pneumonia	2. Chest X-ray-PA/Lateral
3. COPD exacerbation	3. Sputum gram stain and culture
4. Pulmonary embolism	4. Brain naturetic peptide (BNP)
5. Congestive heart failure	5.

1. Opening Scenario

Edgar Furgason, a 47-year-old male, presents to the medical clinic with complaints of nausea and vomiting for the last 48 hours.

2. Vital Signs

BP: 112/60 mmHg

Temp: 99.5° F (37.5° C)

HR: 78/minute, regular

RR: 16/minute

3. Examinee Tasks

1. Obtain a focused history.

2. Perform a relevant physical examination. (Do not perform breast, pelvic/genital, or rectal examination.)

3. Discuss your initial diagnostic impression and your work-up plan.

4. After leaving the room, complete your patient note on the given form.

Are the Vital Signs Stable?

Subjective

Knock; enter. Introduce yourself, and place the first signpost.

"Hello Mr. Furgason, I'm Dr. LaCrosse. I understand you have some nausea today and have thrown up some. Please tell me more about what is going on?"

Transition statement of empathy.

"Hi Dr. LaCrosse. I've been feeling very bad for **2 days** now. I'm just so sick of feeling this way. I've had the flu and throwing up for so long and I need some medicine. I'm nauseated constantly, and I've thrown up over and over. I can't even keep jello down."

"That sounds miserable. I sure hope I can help today because I want to make you feel better as quickly as possible. I'd like to ask a few questions and then do a quick physical exam to find out what might be wrong. I might need to

do a few tests, then I can come up with a treatment plan that I hope will help. Is that ok?"

"Sure."

"Ok. When did this all start?"

"It started **2 days ago**. I **don't know why,** but I got up in the middle of the night, about 4:00 in the morning and just started **throwing up**. I started throwing up and threw up about four or five times. It really surprised me, but I sort of emptied out and then went back to bed. I felt like I had a **fever** at the time, but I just wanted to sleep. My wife got up with me at the time, and by the time I was done in the bathroom, it was time to get the kids ready for school. I have two daughters. So, then she got them off to school and I just stayed in bed. When she left for work, I started throwing up again, and it was just miserable. I just threw up all day that day and stayed in bed."

"Boy, that does sound miserable. Was there any blood in the vomit at all?"

"**No**, no blood but I got to the point of **dry heaving**, you know. Some **brown and green stuff** started coming up after all the food from the night before. It was gross."

"That sounds like a substance your gut makes called 'bile.' Did you take your temperature around that time?"

"Yeah, it was normal—like **98 degrees** at the time."

"Ok. Did you have diarrhea at all then?"

"**No**, not then. The **diarrhea came on later**. Yesterday it started. I started having really loose stools that went to diarrhea. That just made everything worse. It got really watery and gross."

"Was there any blood in that at all?"

"**No**. I just emptied out though. Not much else to say about that."

"Did you have any abdominal cramps or abdominal pain throughout this whole illness?"

"**Yeah**, mostly with the throwing up. My stomach got sore, you know, and hurt. It also hurt when the diarrhea started, but it started when I was throwing up."

"Where was the pain?"

"Right here mainly [pointing to his **epigastrum and left lower quadrant**]. It's not really there anymore though. It was there at its worst but kind of went away."

"Ok. Let's talk about your diet a little bit. What did you have for dinner the night before all this happened?"

"I had the **fish** at a **restaurant** nearby. We go there all the time, it's really good. I don't think it had to do with that place. My **wife had the same thing, and she's feeling fine**. It all came up that morning though."

"Did your wife share your actual meal at all?"

"**Yeah**, actually, she took a few bites of mine. I gave her my mashed potatoes that night, too. She's fine."

> The most common cause of hematemesis after wretching vomiting is Mallory-Weiss tears of the esophagus.

> Assess for others sharing a suspicious meal and ascertain if they're ill as well.

"Ok. So since this came on, have you had anything to eat or drink?"

"The morning it came on, I couldn't even keep water down, it was that bad. I just threw up everything. So nothing all day, but then yesterday I ate some **crackers in the afternoon**. I know you're going to tell me that I should drink more liquids, so I tried that too. I threw up some flavored water last night. I diluted it with about half of regular water, you know. It still all came up."

"Well, diluted electrolyte solutions are good for you if you have a lot of fluid leaving your body, but of course, I don't want to make you sicker. Have you been urinating at all?"

Urine output is an excellent clinical assessment of hydration status; however, patient reliability can be poor.

"Um, I **peed the first day**. I haven't really thought about that. **Not really in the last day**."

"Ok. Are you still nauseated?"

"Oh **yeah**, **I'm still feeling sick**. I feel like I'm totally empty though."

"I'll bet. Do you still have that diarrhea as well?"

"A **little** but that's slowed down a lot."

"During this whole episode, have you had any other problems such as body aches or headache?"

"**Yeah**, I have a **headache** now. It's sort of a dull pain all over. It hurts more when I move my head quickly. I also have **aches all over**. Like my **skin and muscles just ache**."

"Any dizziness or lightheadedness, especially when getting up from a seated position?"

"**No**, not really. Maybe if I get up from sleeping really quickly."

"Have you taken any medications for this?"

"**No**, I haven't taken anything."

"Are you on any regular medications at all?"

"**No**, I take vitamins regularly, but I haven't taken those in a while because I know I would have thrown them up."

"Ok. Do you have any other health issues that are going on?"

"**Nope**, this is it. I've been **trying to lose weight,** but that's all."

"Ok. Have you tried any unusual diets recently?"

"I was on a **soup diet** for about a week; this was **2 months ago**. I quit that though because my friend, who's a nurse, told me to stop."

"Have you had any surgeries in your life?"

"I had my **tonsils out** when I was 13 years old. And when our youngest was born I had an appendicitis 2 weeks before and had to have it taken out. Nothing other than that."

"Alright. Do you smoke or use tobacco in any way?"

"**No**."

"How about drink alcohol?"

"I have a **glass of wine or whatever** with dinner sometimes but not much."

"Did you have alcohol the night before this came on?"

"**Yeah**, I think so."

"Ok. And finally, has anyone else in your family had an illness like this?"

"**No**, everyone else is fine, including my wife. She never gets sick."

Signpost for the Physical Exam

"Ok. I'd like to do a physical exam now, if you don't mind. Just let me wash my hands. It looks like your **vital signs are normal**. I'd like to ask you to roll onto your back…"

Objective

Points for Every Exam:

- Wash hands.
- Comment on vital signs, even if normal.
- Tell the patient where you are going to examine and disrobe.
- Do not repeat painful maneuvers.

Physical Exam:

Perform a focused physical, by system, from the head down.

System	Exam elements	Findings in this patient
Lung	Listen to 6 different areas of posterior lung fields.	Clear to auscultation
Heart	Listen to 4 different areas on the anterior chest.	Regular, rate, and rhythm. No murmurs, rubs, or clicks heard.
Abdomen	Listen for bowel sounds and bruit's. Observe for ecchymosis. Palpate in all 4 quadrants making sure to start with the right quadrants and working toward the sites of pain. Check Murphy's sign and rebound tenderness over McBurney's point. Percuss out the limits of the liver.	Bowel sounds normal. Murphy's sign negative. No rebound tenderness. No hepatomegally. Tenderness to direct palpation in the left quadrants lower > upper. No peritoneal signs. No referral of tenderness.

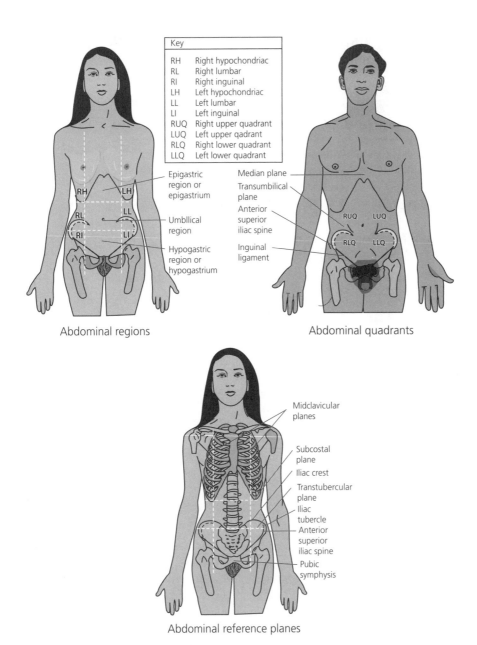

Key

RH	Right hypochondriac
RL	Right lumbar
RI	Right inguinal
LH	Left hypochondriac
LL	Left lumbar
LI	Left inguinal
RUQ	Right upper quadrant
LUQ	Left upper qadrant
RLQ	Right lower quadrant
LLQ	Left lower quadrant

Abdominal regions

Abdominal quadrants

Abdominal reference planes

FIGURE 16.1 Location of abdominal structures by quadrants.

Adapted with permission from Moore & Dalley. *Clinically Oriented Anatomy*, 4th ed. Lippincott Williams & Wilkins, 1999.

TABLE 16.1 Location of Abdominal Structures by Quadrants

Right upper quadrant (RUQ)	Right lower quadrant (RLQ)
Liver: right lobe	Cecum
Gallbladder	Vermiform appendix
Stomach: pylorus	Most of ileum
Duodenum: parts 1-3	Ascending colon: inferior part
Pancreas: head	Right ovary
Right suprarenal gland	Right uterine tube
Right kidney	Right ureter: abdominal part
Right colic (hepatic) flexure	Right spermatic cord: abdominal part
Ascending colon: superior part	Uterus (if enlarged)
Transverse colon: right half	Urinary bladder (if very full)

Left upper quadrant (LUQ)	Left lower quadrant (LLQ)
Liver: left lobe	Sigmoid colon
Spleen	Descending colon: inferior part
Stomach	Left ovary
Jejunum and proximal ileum	Left uterine tube
Pancreas: body and tail	Left ureter: abdominal part
Left kidney	Left spermatic cord: abdominal part
Left suprarenal gland	Uterus (if enlarged)
Left colic (splenic) flexure	Urinary bladder (if very full)
Transverse colon: left half	
Descending colon: superior part	

Clinically Oriented Anatomy. 4th Edition, Moore, K. L, Dalley, A.F. Lippincott Williams & Wilkins, 1999.

Continue to gather information as you do the physical exam. Comment aloud on any real or simulated abnormalities.

Example: *"Does it hurt when I push in here?"*

Example: *"Does it hurt more when I press in or let go?"*

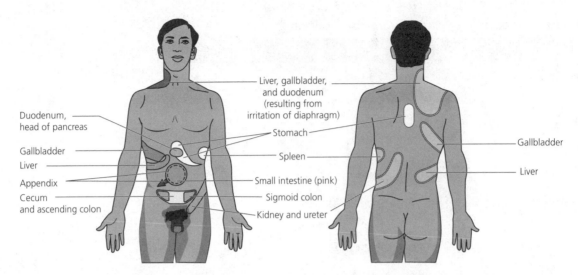

FIGURE 16.2 Pain is perceived as originating in areas supplied by the somatic nerves entering the spinal cord at the same segment as the sensory nerves from the organ producing the pain. Although the areas of pain are not always as shown, they provide clues for the clinician when determining which organ may be affected.

Adapted with permission from Moore & Dalley. *Clinically Oriented Anatomy*, 4th ed. Lippincott Williams & Wilkins, 1999.

TABLE 16.2 Never Root Innervation and Referred Pain Regions Corresponding to Various Organs

Organ	Nerve Supply	Spinal Cord	Referred Site and Clinical Example
Stomach	Anterior and posterior vagal trunks. Presynaptic sympathetic fibers reach celiac and other ganglia through greater splanchnic nerves.	T6–T9 or T10	Epigastric and left hypochondriac regions (e.g., gastric peptic ulcer)
Duodenum	Vagus nerves. Presynaptic sympathetic fibers reach celiac and superior mesenteric ganglia through greater splanchnic nerves.	T5–T9 or T10	Epigastric region (e.g., duodenal peptic ulcer) Right shoulder if ulcer perforates
Pancreatic head	Vagus and thoracic splanchnic nerves.	T8–T9	Inferior part of epigastric region (e.g., pancreatitis)
Small intestine (jejunum and ileum)	Posterior vagal trunks. Presynaptic sympathetic fibers reach celiac ganglion through greater splanchnic nerves.	T5–T9	Periumbilical region (e.g., acute intestinal obstruction)
Colon	Vagus nerves. Presynaptic sympathetic fibers reach celiac, superior mesenteric, and inferior mesenteric ganglia through greater splanchnic nerves. Parasympathetic supply to distal colon is derived from pelvic splanchnic nerves through hypogastric nerves and inferior hypogastric plexus.	T10–T12 (proximal colon) L1–L3 (distal colon)	Hypogastric region (e.g., ulcerative colitis) Left lower quadrant (e.g., sigmoiditis)
Spleen	Celiac plexus, especially from greater splanchnic nerve.	T6–T8	Left hypochondriac region (e.g., splenic infarct)
Appendix	Sympathetic and parasympathetic nerves from superior mesenteric plexus. Afferent nerve fibers accompany sympathetic nerves to T10 segment of spinal cord.	T10	Periumbilical region and later to right lower quadrant (e.g., appendicitis)

(continued)

Organ	Nerve Supply	Spinal Cord	Referred Site and Clinical Example
Gallbladder and liver	Nerves are derived from celiac plexus (sympathetic), vagus nerve (parasympathetic), and right phrenic nerve (sensory).	T6–T9	Epigastric region and later to right hypochondriac region; may cause pain on posterior thoracic wall or right shoulder owing to diaphragmatic irritation
Kidneys/ureters	Nerves arise from the renal plexus and consist of sympathetic, parasympathetic, and visceral afferent fibers from thoracic and lumbar splanchnics and the vagus nerve.	T11–T12	Small of back, flank (lumbar quadrant), extending to groin (inguinal region) and genitals (e.g., renal or ureteric calculi)

Reproduced with permission from Moore KL and Dalley AF. Clinically Oriented Anatomy, 4th ed. Lippincott Williams & Wilkins, 1999.

End of Case

End by explaining you have several ideas of what could be wrong and could cause these symptoms. Tell the patient the first two diagnoses on your differential list and the major tests you'd now like to perform.

Example: *"Mr. Furgason, after talking with you and examining you, there are several possibilities that could be causing your pain that have come to mind. One possibility is that you've contracted a virus that is attacking your gut tract and stomach. This virus may be concentrating on your bowel and be causing your symptoms, which would certainly explain your nausea and diarrhea. Another possible cause is something called diverticulitis, which is a tiny outpouching of the side of the colon wall. What makes this outpouching troublesome is when the end of it gets plugged with something and the whole pouch gets inflamed. This inflamed pouch can be very painful, cause a mild fever, and sometimes produces a small amount of blood in the stool. To test for this, I'd like to get some blood work and a CT scan on you today. There are other possibilities, and those will also be tested for by the CT scan and blood work. There is a small possibility we still won't have the answer after these tests, in which case other ways to look at your lower gut tract may be necessary. I'd like to step out now and set these tests up with my nurse.*

Is there any other aspect of your health care we haven't already discussed? Ok then, thank you."

PATIENT NOTE

History: Include significant positives and negatives from history of present illness, past medical history, review of system(s), social history, and family history.

HPI: 47 y/o male with recent episode of nausea/vomiting and abdominal pain lasting approximately 48 hrs. Nausea and emesis began suddenly and woke pt from sleep and was accompanied by subjective fever. N/V continued over next 24 hrs with no PO intake, including liquids. The next day, the patient reports a trial of crackers and liquid with return of emesis. History of last meal shared by non-ill spouse. Abdominal pain localized mainly to epigastrum and LLQ. Pt denies hematemesis, hematochezia, or fever. Pt reports one glass of wine with dinner at a restaurant the evening before this episode.

PMH: Prior attempts to lose weight on fad diet.

PSH: Cholecystectomy—2 yrs ago; appendectomy.

Tobacco: Denies.

Alcohol use: One drink occasionally.

Meds: Denies.

FamH: Noncontributory.

Physical Examination: Indicate only pertinent positive and negative findings related to the patient's chief complaint.

VS Stable.

Lung: Clear to auscultation. No rhonchi, rales, or wheezes.

Heart: Regular, rate, and rhythm. No murmurs, rubs, or gallups.

Abdomen: Soft, tender in left quadrants lower>upper. No ecchymosis or skin changes, +BSs. No hepatomegally. Neg Murphy's sign. Neg rebound ttp.

Differential Diagnosis: In order of likelihood (with 1 being the most likely), list up to 5 potential or possible diagnoses for this patient's presentation (in many cases, fewer than 5 diagnoses are likely)	Diagnostic Work-up: List immediate plans (up to 5) for further diagnostic work-up
1. Viral gastroenteritis	1. CBC with differential
2. Bacterial gastroenteritis	2. Stool for ova/parasites, white blood cells, culture
3. Diverticulitis	3. Amylase/Lipase, alkaline phosphatase, AST/ALT, Bilirubin (fractionated)
4. Acute pancreatitis	4. Basic metabolic panel
5.	5. CT Scan abdomen with oral and IV contrast.

1. Opening Scenario

Jessica Anderson, an 18-year-old female, presents to the emergency department for nausea and vomiting.

2. Vital Signs

BP: 122/80 mmHg

Temp: 99.8° F (37.7° C)

HR: 88/minute, regular

RR: 20/minute

3. Examinee Tasks

1. Obtain a focused history.

2. Perform a relevant physical examination. (Do not perform breast, pelvic/genital, or rectal examination.)

3. Discuss your initial diagnostic impression and your work-up plan.

4. After leaving the room, complete your patient note on the given form.

Are the Vital Signs Stable?

Subjective

Knock; enter. Introduce yourself, and place the first signpost.

"Ms. Anderson, good to meet you, I'm Dr. Miller. I understand you're having some problems with nausea and vomiting? Please tell me more about it.

"Hi Dr. Miller. Yeah, I've been feeling really bad for the **last couple days**. It started **after a picnic** at my cousin's house. It came on that night. Yesterday it didn't get any better, and I started to **throw up yesterday evening**. It was really bad, and I was very **nauseated**. So, I went overnight and came in today."

"Alright. That sounds like a hard couple of days. Had anyone else at the picnic gotten sick?"

Transition Statement of empathy.

"**No**, my whole family was there. A family reunion, sort of. It was **just me that got sick**."

"Have you also had abdominal pain or just the nausea and vomiting?"

"**Yeah**, my **stomach has been hurting**, too. That's what first started it. The night of the picnic I had to go home because my stomach hurt."

"I'm sorry to hear that. How about diarrhea?"

"**Yeah**, well, the **night of the picnic**, I had diarrhea. Then the **morning after**. The diarrhea went away after that, though. Maybe I just emptied out or something. But then the nausea and throwing up came on."

"Ok. Have you had any fever with this?"

"I've felt **kind of hot** last night. I didn't sweat the bed, but I felt hot. My **whole body aches** though. It's miserable."

"I'm sorry to hear that. I hope we can find the cause of this soon so we can treat it. It's really no fun to be sick. I'd like to talk and ask some questions first and then do a physical exam. After that, I might need to order some tests. That's the best way to tell how to treat you. Does that sound alright?"

"Yeah."

"Alright. Have you taken your temperature at home?"

"**No**, I didn't."

"Have you had any other symptoms other than the nausea, vomiting, brief diarrhea, abdominal pain, body aches, and hot feeling?"

"**Yeah**, I've also been **drinking water like crazy**. I think it's because I had diarrhea and stuff. It's hard to drink with the nausea, but I'm taking small sips. I'm just **thirsty**."

"Has that been the same time period as the other symptoms?"

"**Yeah**, well, maybe it started the day after the picnic or so."

"Have you eaten anything?"

"My mom has given me **toast and some crackers**. I had some **broth**, too. Not much but that's all. It's not that I'm not hungry, it's just that I don't want to throw it up."

"Ok. When you had the diarrhea or vomiting, do you remember any blood in either of those?"

"**No**, there wasn't any."

"Are you still having the abdominal pain now?"

"**Yeah**, it hurts right here [pointing to the **mid abdomen**]."

"Ok. I'll take a look in a moment. On a scale of 0 to 10, 10 being the worst pain imaginable, what rating would you give this pain?"

"Like an **8**."

"Would you say this is a sharp or dull pain?"

"Like, **dull**, it's sort of hurts all over."

"Does the pain radiate anywhere? Such as your back?"

"It's **just in my belly**."

"Do you have any pain in your chest or trouble breathing?"

"**No**, not at all."

> Stating the logical plan up front to a patient who has made a complaint about their illness gives them a focus for your interaction.

"Do you feel like your heart is racing?"

"**No**."

"How about problems thinking straight or any lightheadedness?"

"**No**, I feel like I'm fine as far as that."

"Any problems urinating at all? Burning or going very often?"

"**Yeah**, I feel like I've been **peeing a lot lately**. It's like I'm always in the bathroom. No burning, though."

"Is that during the day or at night?"

"Mostly the day, but I've also been going a lot at night."

"How many times during the day?"

"Maybe **10 or 12 times a day**."

"Ok. When you have to go, does it feel like you really have to go quickly or you might not make it?"

"**No**, not really."

"When you urinate, would you say a lot comes out or just a little?"

"No, it's **a lot**. I mean like, maybe what I usually pee. A **full bladder**."

"It sounds like you have a lot going on, unfortunately. Are there any other symptoms we haven't already talked about?"

"**No**, I think that's it."

"Ok. Have you ever seen the doctor for anything else in your life? Especially anything you've stayed the night in the hospital for?"

"Well, I have **diabetes**. I **take insulin** and stuff. That's another thing; my **sugars have been really high** lately. The doctor told me once that that might happen when I get sick."

"Well, that's true. How high have they been lately?"

"They're usually in the **120 to 150 range**. Maybe a little higher, but then I adjust my insulin. Since this happened they've been **over 200**. I forgot my blood sugar log or I'd show you. This **morning** it was **too high for my meter to register**, it just said 'high' in the window."

"Ok. Have you been taking your insulin throughout this illness?"

"Yeah, I didn't stop because my sugars were high. I would have if they were low, because I'm not eating, you know."

"What's your normal regimen?"

"I take **20 units** of **regular insulin** in the **morning** and **10 units** at **night**. Then I also take **20 units** of **lantus** at **night**."

"How long have you been on that regimen?"

"My doctor and I started adjusting a long time ago and found this works the best. I've been doing this regimen for about **9 months** or so."

"Ok. Is there anything else that I should know about in your past medical history?"

"That's it. Otherwise, I've been pretty healthy. I was really surprised when I found out I had diabetes."

"Yeah, it's a big disease to digest all at once. Most people don't realize how much it changes your life until they're affected by it. I'm glad it was discovered in

If a "unifying diagnosis" seems to be identified in the interview, take note of it, but don't let that cloud your differential.

you, though, because some people go years before they know they even have diabetes.

Have you ever had a surgery?"

"**No**, nothing like that."

"Other than the insulin that we talked about, are you taking any other medicines?"

"I took some **Pepto-Bismol** right after the picnic. I thought that'd help; it didn't. I think I also took two of those chewable **antacid** tablets. That's all though."

"Ok. Are you allergic to anything?"

"**Penicillin**. When I was young, I broke out in a rash when I took it."

"Ok. We'll avoid doing that, then. Do you smoke or use tobacco?"

"**No**, not at all."

"How about drink alcohol or use other drugs?"

"**No**, I don't do that."

"Are you still in school or have you graduated?"

"I graduated in June. Now I'm going to go to university in a month."

"Ok. I'd like to ask some personal questions about your sexual habits and menstrual cycle. Is that ok?"

"That's fine."

"Are you sexually active?"

"With my boyfriend, we've been, you know, intimate, twice."

"Alright. Are you on birth control, or do you use protection?"

"We used **condoms,** but I'm also on the **patch,** Ortho Evra. I put one on once a week."

"Ok. Have your periods been regular or not?"

"**Yeah**, because I'm on the patch they are. When I wasn't on it—I started it about a year ago—they weren't regular."

"Ok. When was your last period?"

"I ended about **3 weeks ago**. "

"Has there been any vaginal bleeding or unusual discharge since then?"

"**No**, nothing."

"Have you ever been pregnant?"

"Oh, **no**, never."

"Alright. Have there been any major diseases in your family?"

"My **dad** has **diabetes**, too. He takes **insulin** like me. I guess that's where I got it from. But otherwise, everyone's healthy."

> Giving warning of personal sexual questions often eases the transition and prepares the patient for these questions.

Signpost for the Physical Exam

"Ok. I'd like to do a physical exam now, if you don't mind. Just let me **wash my hands.** First, I'd like to listen to your lungs…"

Objective

Points for Every Exam:

- Wash hands.
- Comment on vital signs, even if normal.
- Tell the patient where you are going to examine and disrobe.
- Do not repeat painful maneuvers.

Physical Exam:

Perform a focused physical, by system, from the head down.

System	Exam elements	Findings in this patient
General	Note general appearance. Disheveled? Dry mucous membranes?	Dry mucous membranes and ill appearing.
Lungs	Auscultate the posterior and lateral lung fields. Make sure to listen to 6 points on the posterior lung fields.	Clear to auscultation.
Heart	Listen for heart sounds in at least 4 different auscultation points. While auscultating the heart, feel radial and peripheral pulses. Check capillary refill.	RRR no murmurs/rubs/gallops. Peripheral pulses 2+ bilaterally. Capillary refill is prolonged to 3 secs.
Abdomen	Observe for ecchymosis or skin changes. Listen for bowel sounds and bruit's. Ask the patient where their pain is and palpate that area last. Palpate all 4 quadrants, perform Murphy's sign and assess for rebound tenderness over McBurney's point.	Normal appearance. No ascites. BSs somewhat hypoactive, no bruit's. Patient states tenderness is diffuse. Mild guarding in all 4 quadrants and epigastrum. Murphy's sign negative. No rebound tenderness.

Continue to gather information as you do the physical exam. Comment aloud on any real or simulated abnormalities.

Example: *"Do you have pain when I press here?* [while directly palpating the abdomen].*"*

Example: *"Please take a deep breath while I listen to your back."*

End of Case

End by explaining you have several ideas of what could be wrong and could cause these symptoms. Tell the patient the first two diagnoses on your differential list and the major tests you'd now like to perform.

Example: *"Ok, Ms. Anderson, I'm concerned about a possibility that could be happening in your body that's a serious complication of your diabetes. It's called diabetic ketoacidosis, or DKA for short, and it happens when the sugar in your blood gets very high. It's sometimes happens to a person who has diabetes and then gets sick, which causes their insulin requirement to go up sharply. This is a complication I'm not quite sure you're having, and we need to do some tests to find out. I need to take some blood from your vein and some from your artery. That blood from the artery is a little harder to get, and we use a special needle and technique to get it. It may be a little painful but not that bad. Also, I'm going to ask for some urine for analysis but also to run a quick pregnancy test, just to make sure. Another possibility is that you have contracted a bacterial infection of the intestines, which might have come from something you ate at the picnic. That's a little hard to say, too, until we do more testing.*

Is there any other aspect of your health care we haven't already discussed? Ok then, thank you."

PATIENT NOTE

History: Include significant positives and negatives from history of present illness, past medical history, review of system(s), social history, and family history.

HPI: 18 y/o IDDM female with complaints of n/v after eating at picnic 2 days ago. Pt states nonbloody vomiting started approx 24 hrs after meal and was preceded by abdominal pain and nausea. Nonbloody diarrhea noted in first 24 hrs, which then abated. Abdominal pain still present and described as diffuse, dull, and 8/10 intensity. Symptoms accompanied by body aches, subjective fever, and urinary frequency. Denies other urinary symptoms such as dysuria and urgency. Concurrent increase in daily blood sugars noted to go from 120–150s to over 200, with one unreadable finding this AM.

PMH: G0P0. IDDM—treated.

PSH: None.

Tobacco: Denies.

EtOH: Denies.

Drugs: Denies.

Meds: Insulin regimen: Regular 20 units qAM, 10 units qPM, Lantus 20 units qPM. Ortho evra patches. Pepto-Bismol and antacid tablets once during illness.

FamH: Father—diabetes.

Physical Examination: Indicate only pertinent positive and negative findings related to the patient's chief complaint.

VS Stable, respiratory rate 20 bpm noted. Temp of 99.8 F (37.7 C) noted.

Heart: RRR no murmurs/rubs/gallops. Pulses 2+ throughout. Cap refill prolonged to 3 secs.

Lungs: Clear to auscultation bilaterally. No wheezes, rubs, or rhonchi.

Abdomen: Normal appearance. Bowel sounds hypoactive. Mild guarding in all 4 quadrants and epigastrum with mild ttp. No masses. Murphy's sign negative. No rebound tenderness.

Differential Diagnosis: In order of likelihood (with 1 being the most likely), list up to 5 potential or possible diagnoses for this patient's presentation (in many cases, fewer than 5 diagnoses are likely)	Diagnostic Work-up: List immediate plans (up to 5) for further diagnostic work-up
1. Diabetic ketoacidosis (DKA)	1. Electrolytes, BUN/creatinine, glucose
2. Bacterial gastroenteritis	2. Arterial blood gas
3. Viral gastroenteritis	3. Acetone level/Plasma ketones
4. Hyperosmolar nonketotic state	4. CBC with differential
5. Pregnancy	5. β-HCG

18   Nausea and Vomiting

1. Opening Scenario

Edna Burnstein, a 36-year-old female, presents to the emergency room with complaints of nausea and vomiting for the last 48 hours.

2. Vital Signs

BP: 114/70 mmHg

Temp: 100.6° F (38.1° C)

HR: 76/minute, regular

RR: 16/minute

3. Examinee Tasks

1. Obtain a focused history.

2. Perform a relevant physical examination. (Do not perform breast, pelvic/genital, or rectal examination.)

3. Discuss your initial diagnostic impression and your work-up plan.

4. After leaving the room, complete your patient note on the given form.

Are the Vital Signs Stable?

Subjective

Knock; enter. Introduce yourself, and place the first signpost.

"Hello Ms. Burnstein, I'm Dr. Cheyenne. I understand you've had some nausea today and have thrown up some. Please tell me more about what's going on?"

"Hi Dr. Cheyenne. I've been horrible for **2 days**. My body aches, my head hurts, I can't eat…I've had the **flu** and been **throwing up** for so long, and I don't know what it's like to feel normal. I'm nauseated constantly, and I've thrown up a lot. I can't even keep soup down."

"That sounds miserable. What I'd like to do is ask a few questions and then do a quick physical exam to find out what might be wrong. I'll likely need to do a few tests then we can come up with a treatment plan that will tackle this illness. Is that ok?"

Patients might use the word "flu" for anything that gives them generalized myalgias and arthralgias.

"Sure."

"Ok. When did this all start?"

"I think **2 days ago**. I was at work and I threw up about four or five times, after lunch, ya know? It really surprised me, but I sure emptied out. **I felt like I had a fever** then but…whatever. So when I came home, my husband helped me and made me go to bed. He took care of our kids for that time. He took off work so I could stay in bed. I just was taken out. The next day he left for work, and I started throwing up again and it was just miserable. I just threw up all day that day and stayed in bed. That was yesterday, so now I'm here."

"Boy, that does sound bad. Was there any blood in what you threw up?"

"**No**, no blood, but I got to the point of **dry heaving**, my stomach muscles hurt, you know? Some **brown gunk** started coming up; it was pretty gross."

"That sounds like something your gut makes called 'bile.' Did you take your temperature around then?"

"**Yeah**, it was like **99 or 100 degrees** maybe at the time."

"Ok. Did you have diarrhea then?"

"**No**. The diarrhea came later. Yesterday it started. I started having really loose stools that went to really watery. That just made everything worse."

"Was there any blood in that at all?"

"**No**. I don't think so. I never really looked well."

"Did you have any abdominal cramps or abdominal pain throughout this whole illness?"

"**Yeah**, mostly **after the throwing up**. My stomach muscles were sore, you know. The skin around my bottom, you know, got real sore too. I think from the wiping."

"Was there any blood on the toilet paper when you cleaned yourself?"

"Yeah, now that you mention it. Actually, there was some."

"Was it a lot or just a little streak?"

"Well, it was mixed with stool, you know. But, I totally forgot about that. Maybe like a bloody nose. But it was mixed with, you know, stool."

"But, again, you didn't notice any blood in the toilet?"

"I didn't really look much."

"Ok. Where was the pain in your abdomen?"

"Right here mainly [pointing to her **epigastrum** and **right lower quadrant**]. It was there at its worst but kind of went away."

"Ok. Let's talk about your diet a little bit. What was your latest meal before this happened?"

"I had the **steak and seafood at a bistro** in our neighborhood. It was my son's birthday. I don't think it had to do with that place. I was fine into the next day. I skipped breakfast that morning 'cause I was late for the subway."

"Did your husband share your meal at all?"

"Well, **yeah**, he took a few shrimp from mine. He's fine."

"Ok. So since this came on, have you had anything to eat or drink?"

Obtaining a history of recent diet and shared meals can be very important in determining when or if food-borne bacteria are involved.

"The afternoon it came on, I was going to have a late lunch. Like I said, I didn't have breakfast, but that's not unusual for me. Then I just got sick and nauseated. So nothing that day, but then yesterday I tried some **chicken soup** in the afternoon. I threw up **water** earlier than that, so that soup was the first time I've been able to eat at all."

"Well thin liquids are good for you if you've been losing a lot of fluid, but of course, I don't want to make you sicker. Have you been urinating at all?"

"Um, yeah, but it's been much less lately. I think I'm dehydrated, too."

"That's sure possible, as you've lost a lot of fluids without being able to replace them. Are you still nauseated?"

"**I'm getting better;** I feel like I'm totally empty though."

"I'll bet. Do you still have diarrhea?"

"A **little,** but that's slowed down."

"During this whole episode, have you had any other problems such as body aches or headache?"

"Yeah, I have a **headache** now. It's a general **dull pain** all over [pointing to her head]. I also have **aches** in my muscles and skin, you know? Like my skin and muscles just ache."

"Any dizziness or lightheadedness, especially when getting up from sitting?"

"**No**, not really. Maybe if I get up from laying down."

"Have you taken any medications for this?"

"I took some **Pepto-Bismol** in the beginning. At my office. But it came up immediately."

"Are you on any regular medications at all?"

"**No**."

"Ok. Do you have any other health issues that are going on?"

"**No**, this is it."

"I can understand that. I understand you have children. How many?"

"Two boys."

"Have you been pregnant more than that?"

"**Yeah**, I was pregnant in between my kids but had a **miscarriage**. That was 4 years ago."

"Ok. I understand you're married now. Does that mean you're sexually active?"

"**Yeah**."

"And do you use a form of birth control?"

"**No**, not recently. I was going to get on the pill but never came in. We just either use a condom or use the withdrawal method."

"It seems there might be a small chance you could be pregnant then; is that true?"

"I guess so. I hope not, that would be hard timing. But you know, I guess we'd deal with it."

Patients' expectations of your clinical agenda may be wrong; however, don't come out and tell them that. Be gracious about your intentions, but don't argue a point of false assumptions.

If pregnancy is possible, talk briefly about the subject, and ask if there's a reason it wouldn't be possible. This gives the patient a chance to talk about pregnancy-related issues, if present.

"I'm not suggesting you are. It just appears that's one test I'd like to run, ok?"

"That's fine."

"Do you mind if I ask a few more questions about your sexual history?"

"No, go ahead."

"Have you had any unusual vaginal discharge lately?"

"No, not really."

"When was your last period?"

"I ended about a week ago. My periods are about 5 days long. Was no big deal."

"Ok. About how long do you have between your periods?"

"Maybe 28 or 29 days. My periods have been pretty constant."

"Have you had any problems with sexual intercourse or pain?"

"No, it's fine."

"Ok. Have you had any surgeries in your life?"

"I had my **appendix out** when I was 18 years old. And when my youngest was born, I had an **episiotomy**. Nothing other than that."

"Alright. Do you smoke or use tobacco in any way?"

"**No.**"

"How about drink alcohol?"

"I have a **glass of wine** or whatever with dinner sometimes but **not much**."

"Did you have alcohol the night before this came on?"

"**Yeah**, I think so. Two glasses of wine at the bistro."

"Ok. And finally, has anyone else in your family had an illness like this?"

"**No**, everyone else is fine, including my husband. He never gets sick."

Signpost for the Physical Exam

"Ok. I'd like to do a physical exam now, if you don't mind. Just let me wash my hands. It looks like your **vital signs are normal.** I'd like to ask you to roll onto your back…

Objective

Points for Every Exam:

- Wash hands.
- Comment on vital signs, even if normal.
- Tell the patient where you are going to examine and disrobe.
- Do not repeat painful maneuvers.

Physical Exam:

Perform a focused physical, by system, from the head down.

System	Exam elements	Findings in this patient
Lung	Listen to 6 different areas of the posterior lung fields.	Clear to auscultation bilaterally
Heart	Listen to 4 different areas on the anterior chest.	Regular, rate, and rhythm. No murmurs, rubs, or clicks heard.
Abdomen	Listen for bowel sounds and bruit's. Observe for ecchymosis. Palpate all 4 quadrants making sure to ask first about where pain is and examine that area last. Check Murphy's sign and rebound tenderness over McBurney's point.	Bowel sounds normal. Murphy's sign positive. No hepatomegally. Tenderness to direct palpation in the right upper quadrant and epigastrum. No referral of tenderness.

Continue to gather information as you do the physical exam. Comment aloud on any real or simulated abnormalities.

Example: *"Does it hurt when I push in here?"*

Example: *"Does it hurt more when I press in or let go?"*

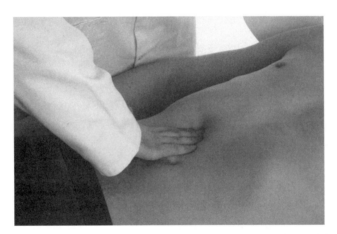

FIGURE 18.1 Murphy's sign. A sign of cholecystitis—pain on palpation over the gallbladder during deep inspiration. Only positive if there is NO pain on the left at the same position.

Reprinted with permission from Thomas & Monahan. *Oxford Handbook of Clinical Examination and Practical Skills.* Oxford University Press, 2007.

End of Case

End by explaining you have several ideas of what could be wrong and could cause these symptoms. Tell the patient the first two diagnoses on your differential list and the major tests you'd now like to perform.

Example: *"Ms. Burnstein, I think you most likely have what's called gastroenteritis. That means the lining of your gut track has become inflamed. When it becomes inflamed like this, the gut can stop doing its job, which is digesting food. It can happen for several reasons, the most common of which is a viral infection, but it can also be caused by bacteria. The difference in these two is that the virus is an infectious agent that can only be treated with supportive measures, whereas a bacteria is a bug we can treat with antibiotics. That's why its important to know the difference, so I'll order several studies to try to tell what's going on with you today. These studies include a blood test and also a stool sample from you for analysis. Now, gastroenteritis isn't the only possibility—just the most likely one. Another possibility is that you may be pregnant, but that doesn't explain all your symptoms; thus, even if you are pregnant, I think there is another probable cause. However, because you have had unprotected sex recently, I'd like to test for that as well. One more possibility is that your gallbladder has some stones in it that are blocking the tube that stretches from it to the intestine. These stones are fairly common, and this could* *explain some symptoms you're having. To investigate this further, I'll want to get a ultrasound of your abdomen. It involves placing a small probe on your abdomen and looking at a screen nearby. It shouldn't hurt but may be slightly uncomfortable. Please allow me to step out to arrange these tests with my nurse so we can get started. Is there any other aspect of your health care we haven't already discussed? Ok then, thank you."*

PATIENT NOTE

History: Include significant positives and negatives from history of present illness, past medical history, review of system(s), social history, and family history.

HPI: 36 y/o female with t2-day history of nausea/vomiting. Vomitis is nonbloody but bilious at times, although decreasing frequency over the last day. Diarrhea also present over the last day and described as watery. Moderate amount of blood on toilet paper, but patient denies overt hematochezia. Infrequent urination and very little PO intake, including fluids, over this illness. These symptoms accompanied by subjective fever, myalgias/arthralgias, headache, and infrequent urination. Last meal consisted of steak/seafood from a familiar restaurant, which was shared by husband without subsequent illness. No other sick contacts.

PMH: Noncontributory.

PSH: Appendectomy, episiotomy.

Tobacco: Denies.

Alcohol use: Mild.

Sexual history: G3P2. Recent unprotected intercourse. Denies dysparunia. Menses approximately 5 days and regular q28 days.

Meds: Pepto-Bismol x 1.

Physical Examination: Indicate only pertinent positive and negative findings related to the patient's chief complaint.

VS Stable. Increased temperature noted.

Lung: Clear to auscultation. No rhonchi, rales, or wheezes.

Heart: Regular, rate, and rhythm.

Abdomen: Soft, mildly tender in left quadrants. No ecchymosis or skin changes, +BSs normal. No hepatomegally. Neg Murphy's sign. Neg rebound ttp. No peritoneal signs.

Differential Diagnosis: In order of likelihood (with 1 being the most likely), list up to 5 potential or possible diagnoses for this patient's presentation (in many cases, fewer than 5 diagnoses are likely)	Diagnostic Work-up: List immediate plans (up to 5) for further diagnostic work-up
1. Viral gastroenteritis	1. CBC with differential
2. Bacterial gastroenteritis	2. β-HCG
3. Pregnancy	3. Stool for ova/parasites, white blood cells, culture
4. Cholecystitis	4. Ultrasound upper abdomen
5. Acute pancreatitis	5. Amylase/Lipase, alkaline phosphatase, AST/ALT, bilirubin (fractionated)

19   Female Abdominal Pain

1. Opening Scenario

Joann Demmer, a 36-year-old female, comes to the emergency room with abdominal pain for 3 days.

2. Vital Signs

BP: 144/90 mmHg

Temp: 99.0° F (37.1° C)

HR: 78/minute, regular

RR: 16/minute

3. Examinee Tasks

1. Obtain a focused history.

2. Perform a relevant physical examination. (Do not perform breast, pelvic/genital, or rectal examination.)

3. Discuss your initial diagnostic impression and your work-up plan.

4. After leaving the room, complete your patient note on the given form.

Are the Vital Signs Stable?

Subjective

Knock; enter. Introduce yourself, and place the first signpost.

"Hi, Miss Demmer, I'm Dr. Simon. I understand you've had some unusual symptoms of abdominal pain. Please tell me more about it."

"Hi, doctor. Yeah, I'm having a lot of pain in my abdomen. It started 3 nights ago and hasn't gone away. It feels almost like really bad **menstrual cramping,** but I can't tell. It's a dull pain that kind of comes and goes."

"Ok. Do you remember what brought it on?"

"Umm, that night, I had **fish** but **nothing out of the ordinary**. I don't think it was the dinner, really, I don't know what it is."

Pain symptoms:
Onset
Provocation
Quantity
Radiation/Relieving
   factors
Symptoms which
   accompany
Timing

"On a scale of 0 to 10, 10 being the worst pain imaginable, where would you place your pain?"

"It's a good **8** right now."

"Does anything make this worse?"

"I've been able to **eat ok throughout this**. I get hungry and am able to keep everything down. There's really **no nausea**. I don't eat as much, but I just don't feel like it."

"Did anyone share that meal with you? Did they have any similar symptoms?"

"Yeah, but everyone's fine. My husband and two daughters ate with me that night and since. **Everyone's ok but me**."

"Where is the pain exactly?"

"It hurts right here [pointing to the lower **quadrants of her abdomen**]."

"Does the pain radiate anywhere?"

Obtain ROS elements throughout the interview.

"**No**, it stays pretty much in the same area. I feel like it's kind of stabbing, you know? Like…stabbing."

"Alright. Is there a time that this hurts more severely? In the nighttime or in the morning?"

Show empathy to patient comments expressing frustration.

"It just **hurts all day**. It really started hurting **worse in the last 6 hours** or so. When I got up this morning, I told my husband how much pain I was in. He said I should come to the doctor, but there weren't any appointments open. I was a little **lightheaded** this morning so he brought me to the ER."

"I know that can be frustrating. Have you taken any medicines to help with the pain? Or done anything that helps it go away?"

"I took some **Tylenol** yesterday, but it really didn't do anything. My husband also gave me one of his pain pills he takes for his knees. **Percocet**, I think. That was last night and that at least helped me go to sleep. Otherwise, nothing."

"Let me ask about your period. When was the last time you menstruated?"

Patients may make self-incriminating statements, such as confessing to taking other's medications. Unless the situation is continually harmful and likely changed by your intervention, don't let these distract you from the point of the interview.

"I haven't had a full period in about a year. I get the **depo** shot every 3 months. I have some spotting from time to time, though. That's never gone away since I started the shot. I had some spotting last night, too. It's not much but it's there, ya know. I've been on the shot a long time, and this pain hasn't ever happened."

"When was your last depo shot?"

"Umm, **2 months ago**, now. I'm due next month."

"Can you tell me more about the actual spotting? Did your discharge look like fresh blood or was it like normal menses?"

"Yeah, it's **like a period**. Maybe a little **darker** but like a period."

"Have you seen any clots in the bleeding?"

"**No**, no clots."

"How many tampons or pads have you used since yesterday?"

"Oh, it's only been **three tampons since last night**."

"Ok. You mentioned you have two daughters. Are they the only times you've been pregnant?"

"Yeah, and my youngest is 10, so it's been a while."

"I know you're married, so may I assume you're sexually active?"

"**Yeah**, we haven't done that in a week though."

"Do you have any problems with having sex? Any pain normally?"

"**No**, although it did hurt a little the last time we did it. It was just kind of uncomfortable, which is weird. It's just kind of weird talking about this."

"I certainly don't mean for you to be uncomfortable with these questions. I'm only trying to get the information that might help diagnose your pain. I know sometimes these questions can be pretty personal, though. If you feel at all uncomfortable with just myself asking these, I'd certainly be able to ask a female coworker come in as well?"

"**No**, that's alright. I just wasn't brought up to talk about this."

"I understand. Would you like to continue?"

"Sure."

"Ok. Other than the blood we talked about, have you had any unusual vaginal discharge?"

"**Nope**."

"Alright. Let me ask you some other questions about what's going on. I understand you haven't had any nausea with this and that you have had a somewhat decreased appetite. Any diarrhea or change in stool consistency?"

"I've been a little **constipated** lately, but that's not that unusual either. I usually go every couple days, but sometimes I go maybe 3 days. I went to the bathroom, number two, **last night** though."

"Ok. Was there any blood in that stool?"

"**No**, it was normal."

"Have you had a fever or other illness recently?"

"**Nope**."

"How about things like breathing problems or chest pain?"

"**No**, spicy food gives me **heartburn,** but I haven't had that in a while. I just avoid spices and tomatoes."

"You said you had gotten lightheaded this morning. Did you pass out or almost pass out?"

"**No**, no. I just felt a little **dizzy** when I got up. It was more like a big **headrush**. My husband thought more of it than I did."

"Do you ever get dizzy like that?"

"**No**. That was the first time really."

"How about any other symptoms, like trouble moving your arms or legs? Eyesight difficulties?"

"**No,** nothing like that. It only lasted about **10 seconds**."

"Have you had any rashes or joint pains recently?"

> Sexual history is important in any female with abdominal pain because of the broad differential.

> Any positive answers in the ROS should be further investigated.

"**No.**"

"*How about headaches?*"

"Almost never."

"*I'd like to ask a little about your past medical history. I understand you've had two children. Were they delivered vaginally or by C-section?*"

"They were both **vaginal**. I didn't have any problems."

"*How about any other stays in the hospital?*"

"**No**, those are the only times. I once was in a **car crash**, about 9 years ago, and was taken to the emergency room in an ambulance but was let go afterward."

"*Do you take any medications?*"

"Like I said, the **Depo Provera**. I take some Tums from time to time and maybe some Tylenol, but that's it."

"*Ok. Have you had any surgeries?*"

"**No**. No surgeries."

"*How about allergies? Do you have any to medicines or any other substances?*"

"**No**, I don't react to anything."

"*Do you smoke? Or drink alcohol?*"

"**No**, I stay away from both of those. I've never done either."

"*Ok. Has anyone in your family had any major diseases like cancer or diabetes?*"

"My mother had **lung cancer** and died at age 72. I never knew my father. I have two sisters that are both younger and are fine."

Signpost for the Physical Exam

"Ok. I'd like to do a physical exam now, if you don't mind. Just let me wash my hands. It looks like your **vital signs are normal** so please let me first listen to your heart and lungs…"

Objective

Points for Every Exam:

- Wash hands.
- Comment on vital signs, even if normal.
- Tell the patient where you are going to examine and disrobe.
- Do not repeat painful maneuvers.

Physical Exam:

Perform a focused physical, by system, from the head down.

System	Exam elements	Findings in this patient
Lungs	Auscultate the posterior and side lung fields. Make sure to listen to 6 points on the posterior lung fields and 1 on each lateral lung field.	Clear to auscultation. No rhonchi, wheezes, or rales.
Heart	Auscultate in at least 4 different areas of the anterior chest. Feel radial pulses, check capillary refill.	RRR, no murmurs, rubs, or orgallups.
Abdomen	Observe the abdomen for periumbilical or flank ecchymosis. Then, listen for bowel sounds and abdominal bruit's. Ask the patient where her pain is and palpate this area last. Palpate the abdomen, asking if she is having pain in each quadrant. Check for masses (comment on lack of them), Murphy's sign, and direct/rebound tenderness over McBurney's point. Comment on findings, such as tenderness affecting other areas of the abdomen or abdominal guarding. Check psoas and obturator signs. No need to percuss organ size in this patient.	The patient appears uncomfortable on palpation of the left lower quadrant. She states that is where her pain is concentrated. Mild muscular guarding when palpating this area. Tenderness does not radiate upon palpation. Negative rebound or ttp over McBurney's point. Negative psoas and obturator signs.
Genital/Pelvic	Deferred	Deferred

Continue to gather information as you do the physical exam. Ask about pertinent aspects of each system as you perform the exams. Comment aloud on any real or simulated abnormalities.

Example: *"Where do you normally get your menstrual cramping when it comes on?"*

Example: *"When you sometimes get constipated, does it hurt in this area?"*

End of Case

End by explaining you have several ideas of what could be wrong and could cause these symptoms. Tell the patient the first two diagnoses on your differential list and the major tests you'd now like to perform.

Example: *"Miss Demmer, your symptoms make me think of several different problems that may be going on in your body. Specifically, I'd like to check for pregnancy, as you're sexually active. I know you're on birth control but there's a slight chance you may be pregnant or have a special type of pregnancy that occurs outside of the uterus called an ectopic pregnancy. I'd like to obtain a pregnancy test as well as some other lab work to evaluate for this. I'd also like to complete an ultrasound on you. The ultrasound will be best performed on your abdomen, but we will also get the best images by looking through your vagina at your uterus and ovaries as well. This test can be uncomfortable but is usually not painful. Before I do those tests, I'd like to do a regular pelvic exam and take some samples of the fluid from your cervix for analysis. This will help me evaluate for another possibility of your symptoms, which includes an infection of your genital tract. That exam is like one you've probably had for a pap smear before. We can do the pelvic exam and the ultrasound at the same time so it will only be a little while you have to be uncomfortable. Please feel free to have a family member present during these exams. There will also be a female nurse here during these as well.*

I have to step out and arrange these things with the nursing staff. Before I go is there any other aspect of your health care we haven't already discussed? Ok then, thank you."

PATIENT NOTE

History: Include significant positives and negatives from history of present illness, past medical history, review of system(s), social history, and family history.

HPI: 36 y/o female with lower abdominal pain for 3 days. The pain started without association to meals and was not accompanied by n/v/d. Pain is characterized as dull, 8/10 and worsening over recent 6 hrs. No radiation, mild decrease in appetite, no accompanying fever. She did take Tylenol without relief and Percocet x 1, which helped with sleep. Lying down reportedly improves pain. Neurologic symptom of dizziness noted on rising from bed this AM but denies LOC or other episodes of same. Positive recent vaginal spotting, which she ascribes to her 1 year history of Depo Provera shots. No chest pain or palpitations. No change in bowel habits, last BM in prior 24 hrs.

Meds: Depo Provera, last dose 2 months ago. Occasional Tylenol and antacid (Tums).

PMH: G2P2 female. Vaginal delivery x 2.

PSH: None.

Smoking: Denies.

Alcohol use: Denies.

Allergies: NKA.

FamH: Mother—deceased, lung cancer; father—unknown.

Physical Examination: Indicate only pertinent positive and negative findings related to the patient's chief complaint.

VS Stable. Elevated blood pressure noted.

Lungs: Clear to auscultation. No wheezes, rhonchi, or rales.

Heart: RRR no murmurs, rubs, gallops. Pulse's normal-radial. Cap refill <2 sec.

Abdomen: Soft. Normal bowel sounds. No abdominal bruit's. No masses. Positive ttp in left lower quadrant. No rebound tenderness. Negative peritoneal signs. Negative psoas/obturator signs. No ttp over McBurney's point. No discoloration.

Back: Negative CVA tenderness.

Differential Diagnosis: In order of likelihood (with 1 being the most likely), list up to 5 potential or possible diagnoses for this patient's presentation (in many cases, fewer than 5 diagnoses are likely)	Diagnostic Work-up: List immediate plans (up to 5) for further diagnostic work-up
1. Ectopic pregnancy	1. Pelvic exam
2. Pelvic inflammatory disease	2. β-HCG
3. Ovarian cyst	3. Chlamydia and gonococchal antigen testing.
4. Spontaneous abortion	4. CBC with differential
5. Diverticulitis	5. Abdominal/transvaginal ultrasound

20   Anterior Knee Pain

---

1. Opening Scenario

David Timmers, a 24-year-old male, comes to the clinic complaining of unilateral knee pain.

2. Vital Signs

BP: 128/78 mmHg

Temp: 97.9° F (37.1° C)

HR: 66/minute, regular

RR: 12/minute

3. Examinee Tasks

1. Obtain a focused history.

2. Perform a relevant physical examination. (Do not perform breast, pelvic/genital, or rectal examination.)

3. Discuss your initial diagnostic impression and your work-up plan.

4. After leaving the room, complete your patient note on the given form.

Are the Vital Signs Stable?

Subjective

Knock; enter. Introduce yourself, and place the first signpost.

"Hello, Mr. Timmers, I'm Dr. Cloke. I understand you've had some knee pain lately. Please tell me more about it."

"Yeah, doctor, my **right knee has been hurting** quite a bit in the **last week**. I can't stand it anymore, so I had to come in to have you look at it. I'm not one for doctors, but this has been hurting."

"Ok. Your right knee… when did the pain come on, and what do you think brought it on?"

"It's been there for about a week. Started at work at the **end of the day** on Monday. I'm a **roofer,** and so I **kneel** all the time. I was up on a project, and it just started hurting. I mean, I get knee pain a lot, you know, a lot. But this just didn't go away like it normally does when I stand up."

Pain symptoms:
Onset
Provocation
Quantity
Radiation/Relieving factors
Symptoms which accompany
Timing

When asking for a pain scale rating, always ask on a scale of 0 to 10, not 1 to 10. Also, always describe 10 as the "worst pain imaginable."

The pain scale of 0 to 10 is a relative scale. Later in the course of disease, the same scale may be used for comparison to rate the effectiveness of treatment.

"It sounds like you're kneeling quite a bit. Did you injure it in any way? Was there a time you accidentally hit it on something?"

"No, actually, that day I **forgot my knee pads** at home. I sometimes do that. But then toward the end of the day I just couldn't work anymore. The next day I did have my knee pads, but that same spot hurt just the same. I didn't actually injure it at all at the time. Now when I even try to jog or exercise I can even feel it."

"Ok. Is the pain sharp or a dull ache? Does it radiate anywhere?"

"Well, it's **hard to describe as sharp,** but it hurts just in this spot [pointing to the anterior knee under his robe]. The pain is just in that spot, **doesn't go anywhere**. It's almost like it's just that spot, you know?"

"If you had to place the pain on a scale of 0 to 10, 10 being the worst pain imaginable, where would you rate it?"

"I'd say about a 6. It hurts pretty bad."

"Alright, does the pain cause you to limp, or has your knee ever given out because of the pain?"

"Well, it does hurt a little when I walk; it comes on more when I'm kneeling on the roof, though. And like I mentioned, it aches when I jog. I used to do that every day, but now I haven't run in few days."

"Ok. Have you done anything that eases the pain?"

"I took some **ibuprofen** yesterday and some **Tylenol** before that. It helped a little, but it still hurts. I can walk but it just makes my job harder, you know."

"I can imagine. Can you tell me if there are any other problems you've had because of this pain? Things like swelling or inability to bend the knee?"

"Well, it **looks pretty red** when I'm done with a day of work, and it feels kind of **warm**. Maybe some **swelling**, too. It feels like I can still move around, and it might be a little hard to bend but…."

"Have you had a fever in the past week?"

"**No**. Otherwise, I've been fine."

"Are there any other joints that hurt as well or just the knee?"

"**No, just the right knee**. Like I say, otherwise, I'm good."

"Ok. I'll take a good look at it in a moment. Have you had any other problems you've had to see the doctor about in your life? Especially anything you've had to stay the night in the hospital for?"

"Not really…when I was 12 years old, I **had my appendix out**. And I played football in high school and **tore my left ACL** up. I did have surgery for that but didn't stay the night. I can't think of anything else."

"Hmmm, you had a left knee injury, huh? Did you ever injure the right one?"

"No, it was **only the left**, and it ended my season my senior year. We were almost done anyway. Ain't like I was star of the team or anything. Never a problem with the right one, though."

"Let me ask a bit about your sexual history, if you don't mind. I ask these questions because, rarely, joint pain in one joint can be a sign of sexually transmitted disease. Rarely, but I'd like to ask a few questions, if that's ok?"

"Sure, fire away."

"Do you have sex with anyone now?"

"I broke up with my last girlfriend **a year ago**. She was the last one. There's been no one since."

"Do you now or have you ever had symptoms of a sexually transmitted disease? Things like burning when you urinate or discharge from your penis?"

"**No**, I've never had that stuff. I've only had sex with five women, and they were all clean."

"Ok. Do you take any medications other than the ibuprofen and Tylenol you mentioned?"

"**Nope**, I don't like to take medications."

"How about supplements—anything like extra protein or creatine?"

"Yeah, I do take **protein**. It's for muscle-building so I can put on some weight. No other supplements, though."

"Ok. How about smoking or dipping? Do you do either of these?"

"I **dip about half a can per day**. On the job site I can't smoke. I've done that for about **2 years**."

"Would you like help quitting?"

"**Nah**, I don't want to try for a while."

"Ok. How about alcohol? Do you drink?"

"I drink about **two to three beers per night**, a **little more on the weekends**."

"How much more on the weekends?"

"Oh, I go out with my friends and drink probably **seven to eight beers**. I don't like liquor, but we just go out to relax."

"I see. Have you ever tried to cut down?"

"**No**, I don't really drink that much, I think."

"Have you ever felt annoyed by someone commenting on your alcohol intake?"

"**No**, my girlfriend didn't like it, but she never annoyed me."

"Have you ever felt guilty because of your drinking?"

"**No**, I don't feel guilty. I don't drink enough for that."

"Ok. Have you ever taken a drink in the morning, like what's called an 'eye opener?'"

"**No**, I've never done that. I don't drink in the mornings."

"Ok. Let me ask a little about your family. Has anyone in your family ever had a major disease, such as cancer, heart disease, or especially any trouble with their joints?"

"My dad's a tax attorney, and he has **high blood pressure,** but he's fine. My mom and him are divorced, and she had **breast cancer** 2 years ago. She had surgery and is on medication now but is alright. Nothing else in my family."

A sexual history may help narrow the possibility of gonococcal-related septic arthritis.

Supplement intake is important in joint pain patients. Protein supplements may induce gouty attacks.

When alcohol consumption is present in excess, ask the CAGE questions:
Cut down?
Annoyed by others mentioning excess drinking?
Guilty?
Eye openers?

Signpost for the Physical Exam

"Ok. I'd like to do a physical exam now if you don't mind. Just let me wash my hands. It looks like your **vital signs are normal,** so please **let me ask you to pull up the bottom of your robe** to look at your knees as you sit there…"

Objective

Points for Every Exam:

- Wash hands.
- Comment on vital signs, even if normal.
- Tell the patient where you are going to examine and disrobe.
- Do not repeat painful maneuvers.

Physical Exam:

Perform a focused physical, by system, from the head down.

System	Exam elements	Findings in this patient
Musculoskeletal	Observe both knees side by side and compare during the exam. Perform Lachman's maneuver, anterior/posterior drawer signs, Apley's compression test, valgus and varus testing, and McMurray testing. Assess for effusion by checking for patellar ballottement and fluid wave.	There is a reddened area over the right knee. No effusion is present but there is moderate soft tissue swelling. The anterior knee is slightly tender in the midline. No instability or ligamentous laxity.
Neurologic	Assess tactile sense of the lower extremities. Test proprioception of knee/ankle/toes. Check deep tendon reflexes, although don't strike the place the patient has pain.	Normal
Skin	Check the area of pain for signs of infection (erythema) or places of skin break.	There is a reddened area around the anterior right knee without signs of skin breaks. No fluctuance or focal induration.

Continue to gather information as you do the physical exam. Comment aloud on any real or simulated abnormalities.

Example: *"Does this maneuver cause more pain?"*

Example: *"Can you show me what makes this pain worse?"*

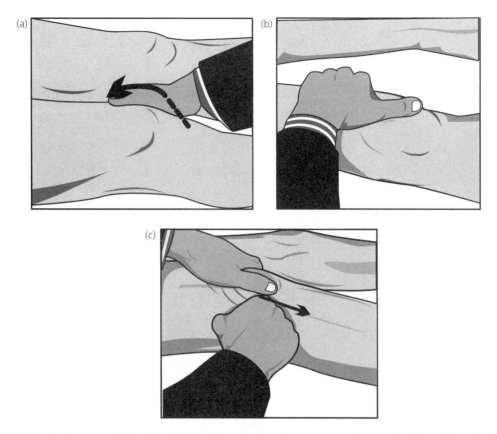

FIGURE 20.1 The bulge test. (a) Stroking fluid proximally into the suprapatellar pouch. (b) Holding the fluid in the suprapatellar pouch. (c) Stroking fluid distally from the suprapatellar pouch.

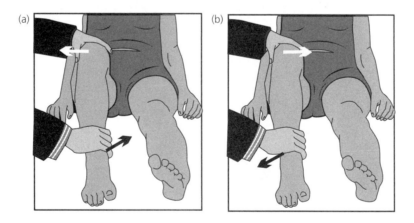

FIGURE 20.2 Assessment of the collateral ligaments. (a) Stressing the lateral collateral ligament: the white arrow represents the force generated by the left hand to stabilize the knee (to prevent its movement). The right hand attempts to move the ankle medially. (b) Stressing the medial collateral ligament.

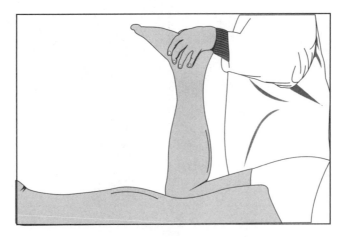

FIGURE 20.3 Examination of the knee with the Apley test.

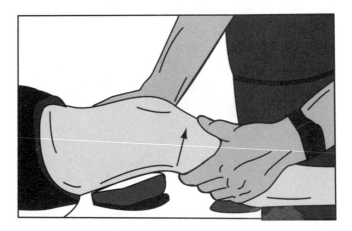

FIGURE 20.4 Lachman's Maneuver.

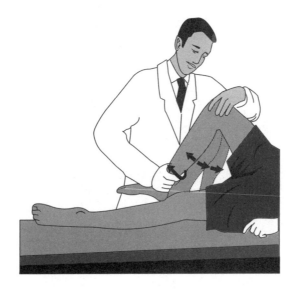

FIGURE 20.5 McMurray's Maneuver.

End of Case

End by explaining you have several ideas of what could be wrong and could cause these symptoms. Tell the patient the first two diagnoses on your differential list and the major tests you'd now like to perform.

Example: *"Mr. Timmers, your symptoms make me think of several different diseases that may be going on. Specifically, this may be a disorder called bursitis, another one called cellulitis, or even a few other things. I'd like to obtain some samples to test for what might be wrong. To test for the cause, we will need both blood from your arm as well as fluid from the space within the knee itself. The test on the knee fluid will require me to insert a needle into your knee joint right here [point to the entry point for aspiration]. This procedure should not be too painful as I'll be able to numb the area before we start. Most people are surprised at how easy it is. I don't think we have time for this today, so I'd like you to come back for the test later, that way I can devote the time that I think this procedure warrants. I also would like to get an X-ray of that knee, if you don't mind. You can do this just before the procedure at your next appointment, too. I would also like you to schedule an appointment for 1 or 2 days after the fluid and blood are taken to discuss your results. Please feel free to get dressed, and I'll have my nurse assist you with those appointments.*

Is there any other aspect of your health care we haven't already discussed? Ok then, thank you."

PATIENT NOTE

History: Include significant positives and negatives from history of present illness, past medical history, review of system(s), social history, and family history.

HPI: 24 y/o male with anterior knee pain x 1 week. He states this pain started after working at his roofing job without knee pads. He states the knee has had pain in the anterior location accompanied by redness and warmth progressive until this appointment. Pain does not radiate, and he denies fever or systemic symptoms. Inconsistent ibuprofen and Tylenol has led to unsatisfactory relief. Symptoms most affect him upon kneeling at work and is rated as 6/10, although some pain is also there on jogging>walking.

ROS: No fever. No complaints of arthralgias in the other joints. Otherwise noncontributory.

Meds: Inconsistent use of ibuprofen and Tylenol

PMH: Noncontributory.

PSH: Left ACL repair—historic. Appendectomy—childhood.

Tobacco: Dipping ½ can per day x 2 years.

Alcohol use: 2-3 drinks/day, 6-7 drinks on weekends. CAGE negative.

FamH: Father—high blood pressure; mother—breast cancer.

Physical Examination: Indicate only pertinent positive and negative findings related to the patient's chief complaint.

VS stable, normal.

Extremities: Right knee examined. Mild erythema over anterior prepatellar area. Moderate swelling. No fluid wave, negative ballottement. McMurray, varus/valgus, Lachman's, and anterior/posterior drawer signs negative.

Skin: Mild erythema over anterior right knee. No ecchymosis. No lymphangitis. No visible skin breaks or rashes. No fluctuance or focal induration.

Neuro: Lower extremity: Strength 5/5 throughout, tactile sensation intact, Reflexes 2+ bilaterally. Right quads reflex differed.

Differential Diagnosis: In order of likelihood (with 1 being the most likely), list up to 5 potential or possible diagnoses for this patient's presentation (in many cases, fewer than 5 diagnoses are likely)	Diagnostic Work-up: List immediate plans (up to 5) for further diagnostic work-up
1. Bursitis	1. CBC with differential
2. Cellulitis	2. Synovial fluid aspiration, fluid analysis and culture
3. Gonococcal arthritis	3. Knee X-ray (weight bearing)
4. Patellofemoral syndrome	4.
5. Gout	5.

1. Opening Scenario

Josh McBerry, a 20-year-old male, comes to the clinic complaining of right wrist pain.

2. Vital Signs

BP: 118/60 mmHg

Temp: 98.5° F (36.9° C)

HR: 48/minute, regular

RR: 12/minute

3. Examinee Tasks

1. Obtain a focused history.

2. Perform a relevant physical examination. (Do not perform breast, pelvic/genital, or rectal examination.)

3. Discuss your initial diagnostic impression and your work-up plan.

4. After leaving the room, complete your patient note on the given form.

Are the Vital Signs Stable?

Subjective

Knock; enter. Introduce yourself, and place the first signpost.

"Hello Mr. McBerry, I'm Dr. Stacks. I understand you've had some pain in your wrist. Please tell me how all this started."

"Hi Dr. Stacks. Yeah, my **right wrist** has been killing me for about a **month** now. I play **baseball** and had a rough game, and after the game it hurt. I guess it's no big deal, but it's just that the pain hasn't gone away and I think it's getting worse."

"Well, we should definitely check this out, I'm glad you came in. Do you remember injuring it in that game?"

"Well, I **don't remember** a specific incident. All I know is that the game was pretty intense, and it got kind of rough. I mean, I don't remember ever really, like, going down and hurting it, but there were a few plays that

> Patients may minimize symptoms in an effort to either gain sympathy or because they don't feel their symptoms warrant your time. You should acknowledge that their symptoms are important and they take center stage in your visit.

it could have happened. I remember that **after the game** it was hurting is all I know. It got kind of **swollen the day after** that, too. That's what I remember. But, you know, it wasn't anything I couldn't handle."

"Do you remember falling down or perhaps sliding into a base during that game?"

"Well, **yeah**, I guess. I was a runner on a play and I had to run into home, and me and the catcher kind of **hit each other,** you know, but it wasn't that big a deal. I was running and he was catching the ball and I **slide on my stomach**, you know, like Pete Rose? And I hit him but it really wasn't that hard. He didn't drop the ball or anything, so that was it."

"Do you remember anything else, like catching the ball with your wrist or even perhaps hitting the ball with the bat, that might have injured it?"

"Um, I struck out twice, and then I hit a ball to center field. It was tied and in extra innings so that's why I remember. I got out, though. But when I hit it, the **bat broke**, you know? I think it was just a weak bat, but it broke it and I dropped the bat because it **hurt my hands**."

"You must be a pretty good hitter. Did the pain start after the bat broke?"

"Well, maybe. That **did hurt** now that I mention it. I can't say for sure, though."

"Ok. When you first noticed the pain, was there any bruising or redness?"

"**No**, like I said, that sort of came on the day after. But it was sore that night."

"When it did get swollen, was there bruising also?"

"**No**, not really. It just hurt mainly. I guess it was a little swollen for a while but not that long really. It hurt more to, you know, drive and **turn the wheel** and stuff. It also hurt to bat but we only had one more game and we ended the season."

"Since then, has the pain gotten worse or better?"

"I'd say it's about **the same**. I guess maybe a **little better** but that's why I'm here. Because it hasn't gotten much better in that time."

"I can understand that. On a scale of 0 to 10, with 10 being the worst pain imaginable, what would you say the pain is right now?"

"Probably a **4**, I guess."

"Does the pain stay all in the wrist, or does it move up your arm or into your hand?"

"It's **all in my wrist**. Right here [indicating the dorsal aspect of the right wrist]."

"Ok. Does anything make the pain better?"

"Well, **not moving it**, maybe. Other than that, I haven't tried anything. I took some **ibuprofen** and some **Tylenol,** but they didn't help much."

"How much of those did you take?"

"I took two of the ibuprofen one day, and I tried two tylenol maybe a couple days later. I'm not big on pills. I don't know, maybe they helped a little."

When striking a ball in baseball, or any sport using a racquet, it's possible that the energy from the force is transmitted to the swinging arms and causes injury.

"Ok. Have you noticed the pain getting much worse during a certain time of day? Perhaps in the morning or evening?"

"**No**, not really."

"Have you ever had pain like this in a joint before or is this the first time?"

"I had a **ligament tear** in my knee 2 years ago during my senior year of high school football. But that was a long time ago."

"Ok. Other than this and the knee injury, have you had any other health problems or injuries you've seen the doctor for?"

"**Yeah**, I've seen the doctor a lot. I **broke my ribs** twice in high school, I had **two concussions** at the beginning of college football, and I **sprained my ankle** a bunch of times. Then there's the knee thing that I got operated on for."

"It sounds like you've had quite an active time the last few years. You mentioned that knee got operated on. Were there any other operations?"

"I had **stitches** in my arm right here [indicating a well-healed scar on his left forearm] and here [indicating a well-healed scar on his left shoulder] from when I used to skateboard. That's it, though."

"Do you take any medications other than the ibuprofen and Tylenol you mentioned?"

"**No**, that's it."

"How about any use of tobacco or smoking?"

"**Nah**, I tried it a few times but never liked it."

"Ok. How about drinking alcohol?"

"I do **my share of drinking**, ha, ha."

"How much is that would you say?"

"About a **six-pack on the weekends** or so. Sometimes more."

"How much more would you say?"

"Well, you know, I'm in college. Ok, so I drink maybe a **six-pack during the day,** maybe then a **few shots** during the night. I usually go out with my friends and get kind of **drunk** on the weekends. But I don't drink all week really."

"Alright. Have you ever tried to cut down?"

"**No**, not really."

"Have you ever felt annoyed by someone mentioning how much you drink?"

"**Yeah**, my girlfriend sometimes harps on me about it."

"Have you ever felt guilty about your drinking?"

"**Nope**."

"Have you ever had an eye opener? I mean a drink early in the morning to help with getting up or to lessen a hangover?"

"**No,** I don't do that. That'd make me sick."

"Ok. Has there been anyone else in your family with any major illnesses?"

"**No,** not at all. My little brother's in track, and my parents are both healthy."

> When evaluating joint pain in the setting of injury, don't forget about other causes of pauciarticular arthritis.

> Screening for alcohol abuse in the young male athlete is especially important, considering the inherent risk factors.

Signpost for the Physical Exam

"Ok. I'd like to do a physical exam now, if you don't mind. Just let me wash my hands. It looks like your **vital signs are normal,** so please let me take a look at your wrist…"

Objective

Points for Every Exam:

- Wash hands.
- Comment on vital signs, even if normal.
- Tell the patient where you are going to examine and disrobe.
- Do not repeat painful maneuvers.

Physical Exam:

Perform a focused physical, by system, from the head down.

System	Exam elements	Findings in this patient
Neurologic	Test for tactile sense of both upper extremities. If doubt exists, test sharp/dull sensation on each fingertip. Evaluate deep tendon reflex and muscle strength.	Normal tactile sense without localization of signs of neurologic impairment. Normal DTRs and normal muscle strength.
Musculoskeletal	Observe both wrists for symmetry or obvious differences. Ask the patient where pain is and palpate the region thoroughly taking care not to illicit pain unnecessarily. Concentrate on the right and start with passive ROM followed by active. Assess flexion, extension, ulnar/radial motion, and rotation. Simultaneously assess strength in these motions.	Symmetric appearance. No areas of notable swelling or erythema. Moderate tenderness to palpation over the dorsal aspect of the wrist. Moderate tenderness on direct palpation of the "anatomic snuffbox." Full ROM, although some pain on extreme ulnar deviation in the anatomic snuffbox.

Continue to gather information as you do the physical exam. Comment aloud on any real or simulated abnormalities.

Example: *"Does it hurt more in this area?* [indicating the anatomic snuffbox of the wrist]."

Example: *"Can you show me what makes this pain worse?"*

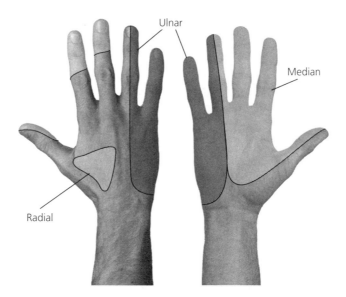

Ulnar

Median

Radial

FIGURE 21.1 Sensory distribution of the major peripheral nerves in the hand. There is a considerable overlap and the small area supplied by the radial nerve may not be detectable clinically.

Reprinted with permission from Thomas & Monahan. *Oxford Handbook of Clinical Examination and Practical Skills.* Oxford University Press, 2007.

End of Case

End by explaining you have several ideas of what could be wrong and could cause these symptoms. Tell the patient the first two diagnoses on your differential list and the major tests you'd now like to perform.

> **Example**: "*Mr. McBerry, it sounds like you injured your wrist in some fashion during that baseball game. To find out how, I'm going to recommend we get some X-rays. These X-rays will be done in several different fashions so I can better see all the bones in there that I have to. Some of the possibilities that I'm thinking of are sometimes caused by what we call a "fall on an outstretched hand." Meaning a fall like this [demonstrating an impact on an outstretched hand]. This can cause a fracture of one or more of the tiny bones inside the wrist and can sometimes cause the symptoms you're describing. I hope to be able to determine that on the X-rays. Another possibility is that you stretched or sprained the ligaments between the bones of the wrist. That can be a serious injury too, as those are important ligaments that hold those bones together. It all depends on what I can determine on the X-rays. Please allow me to step out and arrange these with my nurse so we can get those started.*
> *Is there any other aspect of your health care we haven't already discussed? Ok then, thank you.*"

PATIENT NOTE

History: Include significant positives and negatives from history of present illness, past medical history, review of system(s), social history, and family history.

HPI: 20 y/o male with history of sports related injury to right wrist and subsequent pain for the last 1 month. Pt states he does not recall the injury, although relates a history of several at-risk incidents during a particular baseball game that lead to mild swelling and onset of pain the day after the game. Pain is reported as 4/10 currently and made worse by steering the wheel while driving. He has taken ibuprofen and Tylenol in small amounts without relief. No history of similar pain in the past.

PMH: Fractured ribs, multiple. Multiple ankle sprains. Two concussions. Two areas of laceration and skin suture repair.

PSH: Right knee tendon repair.

Meds: Inconsistent use of Tylenol and ibuprofen.

Tobacco: Denies.

Alcohol use: Socially. CAGE 1/4.

FamH: Noncontributory.

Physical Exam: Indicate only pertinent positive and negative findings related to the patient's chief complaint.

VS Stable, normal.

Neuro: Upper extremities: Strength 5/5 throughout, tactile sensation normal, Reflexes 2+ bilaterally.

MS: Symmetric appearance. No areas of notable swelling or erythema. Moderate tenderness to palpation over the dorsal aspect of the wrist. Full active/passive ROM. Mild pain on ulnar deviation in the area of the "anatomic snuffbox." Moderate tenderness on direct palpation of the "anatomic snuffbox."

Differential Diagnosis: In order of likelihood (with 1 being the most likely), list up to 5 potential or possible diagnoses for this patient's presentation (in many cases, fewer than 5 diagnoses are likely)	Diagnostic Work-up: List immediate plans (up to 5) for further diagnostic work-up
1. Scaphoid fracture	1. Wrist X-rays (PA, lateral, grip, and scaphoid views)
2. Scapholunate ligament dissociation	2.
3. Hook of hamate fracture	3.
4. Radial styloid fracture	4.
5.	5.

22   Joint Pain

1. Opening Scenario

Jim Brownick, a 44-year-old male, presents to the physician's office for evaluation of joint pain.

2. Vital Signs

BP: 144/92 mmHg

Temp: 98.9° F (37.2° C)

HR: 80/minute, regular

RR: 18/minute

BMI: 34 kg/m²

3. Examinee Tasks

1. Obtain a focused history.

2. Perform a relevant physical examination. (Do not perform breast, pelvic/genital, or rectal examination.)

3. Discuss your initial diagnostic impression and your work-up plan.

4. After leaving the room, complete your patient note on the given form.

Are the Vital Signs Stable?

Subjective

Knock; enter. Introduce yourself, and place the first signpost.

"Hello Mr. Brownick, I'm Dr. Stash. I understand you've been having some pain in your joints. Can you tell me about that?"

"Hi, Dr. Stash. Yeah, I've been having a **terrible pain in my knees**. It's gotten **worse** over the last **5 years,** and I just had to come in. It hurts when I **finish my day** of work and come home, the most. I mean, when I'm done moving around the whole day. I think my knees are just worn out."

"Ok. I'm sorry to hear that. You said this has been worse over the last 5 years. Has the pain gradually worsened or gotten worse all of a sudden?"

"Well, it **comes and goes**. I call them **'attacks'** when it gets real bad and my one knee or the other really hurts. It makes it hard for me to walk and it just **hurts** and **gets red** and what not. I mean it's been get-

If possible, always ask open-ended questions—that is, questions that allow the patient to explain in their own words what's happening instead of being answered in a "yes/no" format.

When asking for a pain rating with chronic conditions, both a rating at baseline and at worst is useful.

Regular statements of empathy place the physician and patient on the same side.

ting worse the last 5 years in that it becomes **harder to walk** during these attacks and also it seems like they're **closer together**. Now, I've **always had knee problems**, but now it's becoming more of a problem."

"Are you having an 'attack' now?"

"Yeah, here let me show you."

"I plan to do a full physical in a moment. I'd actually like to first ask you some questions, then I'll take a look. Ok?"

"Sure, no problem."

"Can you describe an 'attack' for me?"

"Yeah, it just takes **maybe a day or so,** and one knee'll start **hurting** and it gets **red** and **painful**. It doesn't happen except maybe **once every few months,** but when it does I'm out of commission for a while. I can walk, but I **don't go to work** or anything. My **grandpa had the same** type of thing; my mom says I got it from him. After a **few days** of pain and taking medicines, it goes away but during that time it hurts."

"That happens about once every few months, huh? How about in between those times—do you still have pain?"

"Oh, **yeah**. My knees are **sore all the time now**. They have been for about **10 years**. A few of my joints are like that but I don't really mind. I know I'm a big person, and that's just part of life."

"On a scale of 0 to 10, 10 being the worst pain imaginable, where would you rate this pain in between these attacks and then during one?"

"If it's bad, I'd say an **8** out of 10. In between times, maybe just a **2** or so. I'm never pain-free, but then I'm not crippled and laying in bed all day either."

"I understand. Have you ever seen a doctor for this pain?"

"Yeah, I've seen **several doctors** over the years. I had one take some **X-rays** a few years back, and he said he wanted me to lose weight and come back. I tried but didn't ever lose the weight. I was on a diet and doing ok, but the weight never really came off. Anyway, the doctors have prescribed me a few medicines. I only still take the pain medicine, now."

"Do you remember those medications?"

"I remember the one I'm on, is called **celecoxib**. I don't recall the others, but I don't take them anyway."

"That's ok. Have you ever had surgery, or has anyone taken a fluid sample from your knee?"

"**No**, I never have had surgery. I know that's what might be coming down the road, though. And no, no one's ever taken fluid from me. That sounds painful. **I hate needles**."

"Well, I understand not liking needles. I don't like them either. Sometimes, that's what's needed to help you, though. If I have to do it later to diagnose you, I'll try to make sure it's as painless as possible. Have you ever seen a doctor when your knees get really bad?"

"I try to **stay at my house** if that happens. I can tell you that it hurts so bad that I don't want to go out. I don't think any doctor has actually seen my knee when it's bad."

"Ok. Do you ever get a fever with this?"

"**No**. Otherwise, I'm alright."

"Have you gotten other problems when your knees flare up, such as aches or pain in your other joints?"

"It's only really in my knees. My **hands hurt sometimes**, though. I mean, I have times when my hands just hurt, too, but they **don't get red and swollen like my knees**, you know."

"Are you able to use your hands when they get bad?"

"Oh, **yeah**. I can always use my hands."

"Do these two 'attacks' tend to happen together—your knees and hands?"

"**No**, the knees can happen almost anytime. The hands, it just doesn't matter, either. But my hands really don't have the bad attacks. It seems like just a dull ache in them sometimes."

"Ok. Getting back to your knees, does the pain radiate anywhere like down your calf or up your legs?"

"**No**, it just hurts in my knee. **Only one knee** really has any problem at a time, though. They almost never go bad at the same time. I mean, they both hurt all the time, sort of a baseline, but an **'attack' only happens to one at a time**."

"Ok. I think you said earlier that when you aren't having an 'attack,' your pain is always there. Is it worse during the day or in the evening?"

"It's worse **after being on my feet all day**. I work in a bakery, in a big factory, you know, and I'm on my feet all day long. When I get done, sometimes everything hurts. But I've done that for years."

"Ok. Does anything else make it worse or bring on more 'attacks?'"

"**No**, not really. Just working hard."

"Does anything make it better, such as rest? Or ice packs?"

"I've tried those ice packs when I get an 'attack.' I guess **they help** somewhat. It makes me feel better anyway. The **celecoxib** works pretty well, too. Before I took that, I had more pain."

"Ok. What other medicines are you on?"

"I take two **blood pressure medicines**. One is **HCTZ** and the other is **ramipril**. I also have **diabetes** and take **metformin** for that. I'm trying to **quit smoking,** so I'm on the **nicotine patches,** too. I've cut down to about 10 cigarettes a day now. That's all."

"How long have you smoked?"

"Oh, about **20 years** now. It's been a **pack a day** up until I started the patches. They're helping me with it."

"That's great. Congratulations on that progress with smoking! So, how long have you been taking that blood pressure medicine called HCTZ?"

"I've been on that for about **7 or 8 years**. The other one I started last year."

"So, to sum up your health problems, it sounds like you have knee pain, high blood pressure, diabetes, and smoking. Is there anything else you've seen the doctor for in the past?"

Don't be afraid to return to the chief complaint for clarification in the middle of the interview. Delineate the details as much as possible.

Never miss an opportunity to congratulate a patient on stopping or cutting down on cigarettes.

"I've seen the doctor for my **weight** too. I've tried a few kinds of diets but they never really stick."

"That can be frustrating. I know that losing weight is a very hard thing to do, and it's also very hard to keep the weight off. It is something that can really help your overall health, though, so I encourage you to keep trying. Have you ever had any surgeries?"

"**No**, I've never had surgery."

"Do you drink alcohol?"

"Usually some **wine with dinner**. I'm one of those wine lovers, you know. I really like it and so have some with dinner every night."

"How much do you have?"

"Oh, about **half a bottle**. That's about two glasses."

"Have you ever tried to cut down?"

"**No**, I love it too much."

"Do you ever feel guilty for drinking that much?"

"**No**, I don't think it's too much, honestly."

"Have you ever felt annoyed with someone else talking about your drinking?"

"**No**, not really."

"Have you ever woken up and had an 'eye opener,' or a drink to get you going in the morning?"

"**Nope**, I don't drink in the morning."

"Please allow me to ask a few questions about your sexual history. Are you in a sexual relationship now?"

"**Yeah**, you could say that."

"Is the relationship monogamous?"

"Well, my **girlfriend** and I have been together about **4** months. It's not really that exclusive, but it's getting there."

"Ok. Have you ever had a sexually transmitted disease before?"

"**No**. I've had probably **20 or so women** in my life. I guess I've been lucky."

"Do you ever have discharge from your penis or burning when you urinate?"

"**No**, not at all."

"Ok. Does anyone in your family have any major diseases?"

"The **men** in my family have also been **big**. My **dad** had **diabetes** all his life. He **died** 2 years ago from a **blood clot in his lung**. My mom is still around, and my brother is taking care of her, but she still lives alone. My **brother** has **diabetes**, too. Like I mentioned earlier, my **grandpa** had **joint problems,** but that's all I know because he died a long time ago, and I never really talked to him about it."

> When moderate alcohol consumption is discovered, ask the CAGE questions.

> Signposting the sexual history prepares the patient for personal questions and eases possible tension in the interview.

Signpost for the Physical Exam

"Ok. I'd like to do a physical exam now, if you don't mind. Just let me **wash my hands.** Please let me ask you to show me your hands…"

Objective

Points for Every Exam:

- Wash hands.
- Comment on vital signs, even if normal.
- Tell the patient where you are going to examine and disrobe.
- Do not repeat painful maneuvers.

Physical Exam:

Perform a focused physical, by system, from the head down.

System	Exam elements	Findings in this patient
Upper extremities	Check ROM and flexibility of shoulder, elbow, and hand joints. Look for joint nodules, inflammation, swelling, or deformity.	Normal exam
Lower extremities	Compare the affected knee with the unaffected side. Start with the general appearance, then feel for pulses, warmth, tenderness, and ROM of the knees. Check for joint effusion by pattelar ballotment. Milk any fluid proximally, and check for the presence of a fluid wave. Check for popliteal, femoral, or inguinal lymphadenopathy. Assess joint stability with drawer signs, Lockman's maneuver, Apley's test, McMurray's test, and varus/valgus testing.	Left knee erythema noted. Moderate effusion noted by ballotment of the patella and fluid wave positivity. ROM: flexion limited by fluid pressure in the knee, extension normal. Pulses, including popliteal, posterior tibial, and dorsalis pedis, normal. No palpable lymphadenopathy. Stability maneuvers, including varus/valgus, anterior/posterior drawer signs and Lockman's, normal. Negative McMurray's and Apley's tests.

Continue to gather information as you do the physical exam. Comment aloud on any real or simulated abnormalities.

Example: *"When I move your fingers like this, does it cause pain?"*

Example: *"Is it painful to walk right now?"*

End of Case

End by explaining you have several ideas of what could be wrong and could cause these symptoms. Tell the patient the first two diagnoses on your differential list and the major tests you'd now like to perform.

Example: *"Mr. Brownick, from talking with you and examining your knee, there are a few possibilities that may be causing the pain you're having. One possible cause is something called osteoarthritis, which is the wearing down of the cartilage between the bones in your knees that can cause pain. That's more likely for the pain that you describe as always being present but is more unlikely to be causing your attacks. I'll have to obtain an X-ray to tell if that's the case, though. The flare-ups of pain might be caused by other processes. There are several arthritis types that have to do with your body's metabolism of a substance called uric acid. The problem is that sometimes the uric acid can build up in your joints and actually form crystals that cause a period of pain and inflammation. Those diseases are called gout and pseudogout, which is very similar to gout. I know you said you hate needles, but the best way to tell if that's happening is by extracting some of that joint fluid with a needle and having the lab analyze it for us. It's a minor procedure and one I can do right here in the office. I'll be numbing up the skin where I put the needle, and it should make the procedure much more comfortable. There are some* *other possibilities as well, which I'd also like to test for by getting some blood from you today. I'd like to step out and have my nurse come in to prepare what is needed for the lab tests and X-rays.*

Is there any other aspect of your health care we haven't already discussed? Ok then, thank you."

PATIENT NOTE

History: Include significant positives and negatives from history of present illness, past medical history, review of system(s), social history, and family history.

HPI: 44 y/o obese male with bilateral knee pain for >5 years. Pain has constant baseline of 2/10 knee pain with 'attacks' involving redness, inflammation, and swelling and increase in pain to 8/10. Attacks occur unilaterally about 1x/few months lasting several days. Previous evaluation involved X-rays only, which are unavailable. Symptoms of joint pain also occur in hand joints, occasionally, but don't involve a flare-up pattern. He denies other systemic symptoms, including fever, body aches. Sexual history is positive for current nonmonogamous relationship although no current symptoms or history of STDs.

PSH: None.

Tobacco: Currently ½ ppd; 20 pack-years.

EtOH: Approx ½ bottle of wine per day. CAGE questions negative.

Meds: HCTZ, ramipril, metformin.

FamH: Father—deceased, PE, diabetes; brother—diabetes; grandfather—similar painful knee problems.

Physical Examination: Indicate only pertinent positive and negative findings related to the patient's chief complaint.

VS Stable. BP elevated and BMI: 34 kg/m² noted.

Upper extremities: Hands: bilaterally normal ROM, motor strength, and appearance. No signs of erythema or nodules.

Lower extremities: Left knee erythema noted. Moderate effusion present by ballotment of the patella and fluid wave positive. ROM: flexion limited by fluid pressure, extension normal. Pulses including popliteal, posterior tibial, and dorsalis pedis normal. No palpable lymphadenopathy. Stability maneuvers including varus/valgus, anterior/posterior drawer signs, Lockman's normal. Negative McMurray's and Apley's tests.

Differential Diagnosis: In order of likelihood (with 1 being the most likely), list up to 5 potential or possible diagnoses for this patient's presentation (in many cases, fewer than 5 diagnoses are likely)	Diagnostic Work-up: List immediate plans (up to 5) for further diagnostic work-up
1. Gout	1. Weight-bearing knee X-rays
2. Pseudogout	2. Knee aspiration with synovial fluid analysis for gram stain, culture, cell differential, and crystal refraction
3. Osteoarthritis	3. CBC with differential
4. Rheumatoid arthritis	4. Rheumatoid factor
5. Infective arthritis	5.

1. Opening Scenario

Joshua Clusky, a 21-year-old student, presents with complaints of lower back pain.

2. Vital Signs

BP:	123/65 mmHg

Temp:	98.9° F (37.1° C)

HR:	42/minute, regular

RR:	12/minute

3. Examinee Tasks

1. Obtain a focused history

2. Perform a relevant physical examination. (Do not perform breast, pelvic/genital, or rectal examination)

3. Discuss your initial diagnostic impression and your work up plan.

4. After leaving the room, complete your patient note on the given form.

Are the Vital Signs Stable?

Subjective

Knock, enter. Introduce yourself and place the first signpost.

"Hello, Mr. Clusky, I'm Dr Stagg, I understand you've been having some back pain, can you tell me more about it?"

"Yeah, doctor, it came on when **I was playing football** about **a week ago**. It was a rough game and I was tackled a few times and noticed it hurt but nothing out of the ordinary. When I was playing I remember specifically a hit that started the pain but I was able to get up and "shake it off". I got hit a few more times after that and it really hurt but nothing to take me out of the game, you know. Then **after the game**, it started hurting really bad and I took some **Motrin** and went to bed. In the morning, I got up and it still hurt and it's been painful ever since."

Pain symptoms:
Onset
Provocation
Quantity/Quality
Radiation/Relieving
factors
Symptoms which
accompany
Timing

Back pain "Red Flag"
symptoms:
Fever
Weight loss
Loss of bowel/bladder
control
Saddle anesthesia
Loss of sensory/motor
control

"Alright, I understand it was a week ago, but specifically, how many days?"

"Well, actually it was Saturday, so **six days**."

"Has anything hurt your back since then? Does any movement or activity provoke more pain?"

"Well, I really haven't done much because, ya know, my back's hurting. When I'm **done with the day** I feel tired and that's really when it hurts the most. Otherwise it feels a little better when I lie down and sit but if I sit too long, it starts to hurt again."

"Ok, is there anything that relieves it then?"

"Like I said, the **Motrin helped** right after the game. I've also taken some Tylenol and Naproxen since then. They sort of help but it still hurts. I've tried some **hot packs** at night, too, but I don't really notice a whole lot of improvement. I feel like the hot packs just make the area feel better, but the pain's still there."

"Yeah, does the pain stay in one spot or does it radiate to another place? Such as your legs?"

"At first it did, when I came off the field after the game it hurt bad enough that it felt like it went **down my leg**. Sort of **down my butt then around to the front somewhat**. Since then, I guess, it might radiate down the back **of my leg** when it's really bad."

"Both legs or just one leg?"

"It feels like the **left** one. I don't get the pain down the right one."

"How about on a scale of 0 to 10, 10 being the worst pain imaginable, where would you place the pain?"

"After the game, I'd definitely say a 10, but since then maybe a **7 or 8**. It hurts bad."

"Is it a sharp pain, a dull ache, electric shocks? What would you say it feels like?"

"It's like an **ache** most of the time. But sort of sharp in the back itself. When it wraps around my leg, it just aches. Not electric shocks, though."

*"Ok, are there any other accompanying symptoms, such as swelling or **especially losing control of your bladder or bowels?**"*

"**No**, no, nothing like that. I can't see it but I don't think there's swelling."

*"Alright, let me ask you about some other symptoms. Have you had a **fever** or experienced any **weight loss** recently?"*

"**No**, neither."

*"How about trouble **feeling your legs or moving them**, especially when you walk?"*

"**No**, that's all fine."

*"Any **numbness** around your **genital or butt area**? Something you might notice when you sit down."*

"**No**, none. That's fine, too."

"Ok, let me ask about some other symptoms, have you had any headaches with this injury? Or neck pain?"

"**Nope**"

"*Ok, how about problems with any other pain in your body?*"

"**No**, I'm pretty healthy otherwise."

"*Any problems breathing or with trouble eating or going to the bathroom?*"

"**Nope**"

"*Alright, tell me about anything else you've seen the doctor for. Have you ever spent the night in the hospital or gone to the emergency room?*"

"Yeah, I've been to the ER a few times. I **hit my head** while skateboarding about 6 months ago and came to get checked out. I didn't hurt anything serious but they kept me over night "for observation". I've also gotten **stitches in my right knee** a few years ago. I also have seen my regular doctor for what he calls **Chlamydia**. He gave me a shot and some pills and no problems since. I haven't been back to see him though."

"*Ok, are you still taking those pills?*"

"**No**, this was about 3 months ago. I finished them all."

"*Ok, I know you mentioned you took some Motrin after the game, are you taking any other medications right now?*"

"**No**, I haven't taken anything since then."

"*Alright, do you smoke or dip tobacco?*"

"**No**, I did try dipping a long time ago but hated the taste. Never did it again."

"*How about alcohol, do you drink?*"

"**No** I don't drink."

"*Any other drugs like marijuana or especially anything you would inject?*"

"Oh **no**, I've never done that."

"*Ok, has there been any major diseases in your family? Especially in your parents or siblings?*"

"My mom had her female organs taken out a few years ago for something called "**fibroids**" and my dad **smokes**. I think he has **diabetes,** he takes pills, too. Otherwise everyone else is healthy."

Signpost for the Physical Exam

"Ok, I'd like to do a physical exam now if you don't mind. Just let me wash my hands. It looks like your **vital signs are normal** so please **let me ask you to stand up and pull up the back of your shirt for me…**"

Objective

Points for Every Exam:

- Wash hands
- Comment on vital signs, even if normal
- Tell the patient where you are going to examine and disrobe
- Do not repeat painful maneuvers

Physical Exam:

Perform a focused physical, by system, from the head down.

System	Exam elements	Findings in this patient
General	Mannerisms seem normal and calm.	Medium build. Not overweight or obese.
Back	Observe for erythema, swelling, deformity, or spasm in the upright and sitting positions. Ask the patient to point to the maximum area of pain-avoid that area at first then palpate it last. Note ishial spine relative height. Complete ROM maneuvers including flexion, extension, lateral, and rotation while communicating with the patient to determine the most painful maneuvers or radiation of pain. Complete ipsi-lateral and contralateral leg raise testing and FABER testing.	The patient points to approximately the L4 level stating pain is unilateral. Palpation of midline spinous processes in the lumbar area produces tenderness. Palpation of the left paraspinal area also produces tenderness. Flexion is somewhat limited by pain, extension is moderately limited. Rotation is normal and lateral ROM is limited on the left side. No reported radiation of pain. The left ischial spine appears higher than the right. Straight leg raise testing is negative. Negative FABER tests.
Neurologic	Perform tactile sense of the lower extremi-ties as well as lower extremity proprioception and sharp/dull testing. Perform deep tendon reflexes bilaterally. Assess motor strength and gait including heel walk and toe walk. Rectal tone is not needed in this case.	Normal motor and sensation throughout. Symmetric DTR's. No pathologic clonus. Gait normal.

Continue to gather information as you do the physical exam. Comment aloud on any real or simulated abnormalities.

Example: *"Does bending forward or leaning back cause an increase or decrease in pain?"*

Example: *"Can you show me where the pain radiated after the game?"*

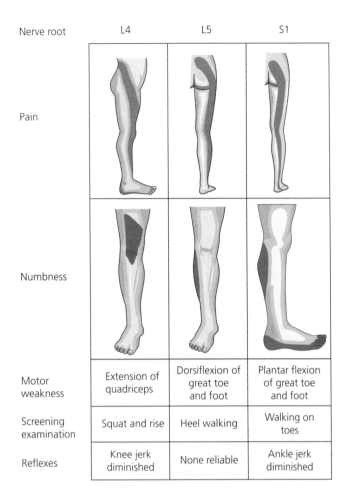

Nerve root	L4	L5	S1
Pain			
Numbness			
Motor weakness	Extension of quadriceps	Dorsiflexion of great toe and foot	Plantar flexion of great toe and foot
Screening examination	Squat and rise	Heel walking	Walking on toes
Reflexes	Knee jerk diminished	None reliable	Ankle jerk diminished

FIGURE 23.1 Testing for lumbar nerve root compromise.

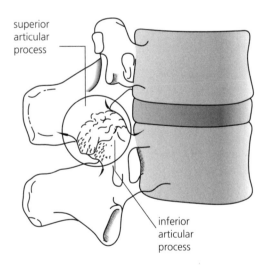

FIGURE 23.2 Fixation of the articular processes.

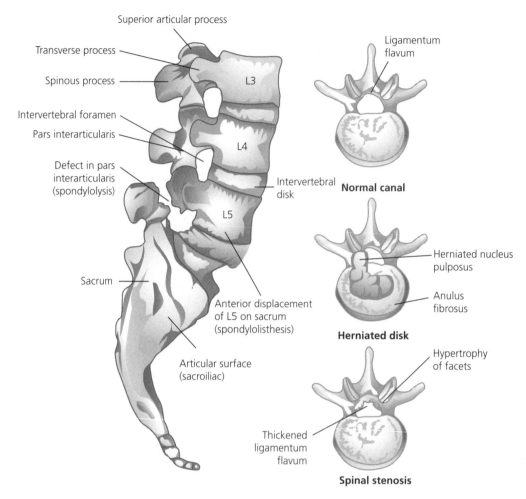

Labels in figure:
Superior articular process
Transverse process
Spinous process
Intervertebral foramen
Pars interarticularis
Defect in pars interarticularis (spondylolysis)
L3
L4
L5
Intervertebral disk
Sacrum
Anterior displacement of L5 on sacrum (spondylolisthesis)
Articular surface (sacroiliac)

Ligamentum flavum
Normal canal

Herniated nucleus pulposus
Anulus fibrosus
Herniated disk

Hypertrophy of facets
Thickened ligamentum flavum
Spinal stenosis

FIGURE 23.3 Herniated disk, annulus fibrosus.

End of case

End by explaining you have several ideas of what could be wrong and could cause these symptoms. Tell the patient the first two diagnoses on your differential list and the major tests you'd now like to perform.

Example: *"Mr. Clusky, after examining you and hearing about your pain, I've come up with several different problems that may be causing it. I think this back pain is most likely due to acute spasm, which come from the muscles in your back being strained causing them to tighten up in a manner beyond your direct conscious control. But, as is commonly the case, only one side of the back has had this reaction which causes the typical pain you're experiencing. A less likely possibility, due to that rough football game, is a fracture of the bony part of your back called a vertebra. I do think this is less likely, however, I will want to obtain an x-ray today to check for this. Low back pain due to local spasm, the most likely possibility here, sometimes lasts for days to weeks and has an association with inflammation in that area. For this disease, medications that both reduce inflammation in your body as well as work to relax your muscles may help. I'd like to try these today. Most back pain of this cause will go away on its own without use of modalities like surgery or local injection. However, if this pain doesn't subside in the period of four to six weeks, please come back for another evaluation. Today, I'll have my nurse refer you to the x-ray department while I obtain your prescriptions.*

Is there any other aspect of your healthcare we haven't already discussed? Ok then, thank you."

PATIENT NOTE

History: Include significant positives and negatives from history of present illness, past medical history, review of system(s), social history, and family history.

HPI: 21 y/o male c/o low back pain x 6 days. Pain started after repeated traumatic events while playing football and was first accompanied by severe symptoms radiating down the left leg and wrapping anteriorly to the thigh region. Pain upon injury was 10/10 but has decreased to 7-8/10 since initial injury. Now pain is sharp in the back but dull as it wraps around the leg anteriorly. The patient states he has tried ibuprofen and Tylenol as well as local hotpacks with minimal relief. The patient denies fever, weight loss, saddle anesthesia, bowel/bladder dysfunction, or loss of motor control.

PMH: Chlamydia. Closed head injury.

PSH: Suture placement right knee-historical.

Tobacco: Denies

Alcohol use: Denies

FamH: Father smokes and has diabetes. Mother s/p hysterectomy for fibroids.

Physical Examination: Indicate only pertinent positive and negative findings related to the patient's chief complaint.

VS Stable, normal.

Back: No focal erythema/swelling, Flexion limited by pain to approx 60 degrees, Extension limited to approx 20 degrees. Mild TTP over L4-L5 spinous processes. Upright ischial spine height discrepancy, left higher than right approximately 2 cm. Ipsilateral and contralateral straight leg raises negative, bilaterally. FABER test negative, bilaterally.

Neuro: Lower extremity: Strength 5/5 throughout, tactile sensation intact, Reflexes 2+ bilaterally. Proprioception normal, bilaterally. Sharp/dull normal. Heal walk and toe walk normal.

Differential Diagnosis: In order of likelihood (with 1 being the most likely), list up to 5 potential or possible diagnoses for this patient's presentation (in many cases, fewer than 5 diagnoses are likely)	Diagnostic Workup: List immediate plans (up to 5) for further diagnostic workup
1. Paraspinal muscle spasm	1. Plain lumbar X-ray, PA, oblique, and lateral
2. Vertebral fracture	2.
3. Intervertebral disc herniation	3.
4. Spondylosis	4.
5. Ankylosing spondylitis	5.

1. Opening Scenario

Mark Shuman, a 73-year-old male, presents to the physician's office with complaints of lumbar back pain for the last 3 weeks.

2. Vital Signs

BP: 140/81 mmHg

Temp: 98.0° F (36.7° C)

HR: 72/minute, regular

RR: 12/minute

3. Examinee Tasks

1. Obtain a focused history.

2. Perform a relevant physical examination. (Do not perform breast, pelvic/genital, or rectal examination.)

3. Discuss your initial diagnostic impression and your work-up plan.

4. After leaving the room, complete your patient note on the given form.

Are the Vital Signs Stable?

Subjective

Knock; enter. Introduce yourself, and place the first signpost.

"Hello Mr. Shuman, I'm Dr. Searles. I understand you're having some back pain. Can you tell me more about it?"

"Hi, Dr. Smith, yeah, I've been having this pain here in my back for a long time now. It's been hurting me real bad **at night**. So, I wanted to come get checked out."

"Alright. Where in your back is this pain?"

"It's down here, down in the **lower back** [pointing to the lumbar area]."

"Ok. Let me take a look in a moment. I'd just like to ask some questions first, if you don't mind. Have you ever had a pain like this?"

"Oh, **sure**. I'm a retired forest service worker. I used to cut trails all my life. I also used to be in the Navy. I know back pain real well. This **hurts like that used to**. I just don't know, though, because I **haven't done anything to bring it on** this time. I don't remember injuring it or hurting it. I thought it'd go away, you know, if I waited long enough. It hasn't, though."

"Alright. Is this pain radiating anywhere, such as down your legs?"

"**Yeah**, it does go down my **right leg**, now that you mention it. Actually, it kind of **wraps around the front of my thigh** right here [pointing to a posterior, lateral, anterior distribution]. My leg **aches at night** and starts with this pain up here in my back."

"It seems like that would be painful. Do you ever have a loss of control over that or the other leg?"

"**No**, I've not had that problem. I can still get around fine."

"Ok. On a scale of 0 to 10, 10 being the worst pain imaginable, where would you put this pain?"

"Well, like I said, I was in the forest service and had a lot of accidents. A little back pain I can handle. It's about a **4**."

"And is this a dull pain or sharp, where it originates in the back?"

"Well, it starts **right there in the one spot**. Right here, I can point to it every time. The pain is always in that spot so I'd say **sharp**, right there [pointing to the lumbar region of his back]."

"Alright. Let me ask you to think back to the first time you felt it. I know you said there wasn't an accident or straining, but what were you doing at the time?"

"Well, let me think…I think I just **woke up with it about 3 weeks ago**. It just came on one morning. Nothing out of the ordinary."

"And has the pain increased or decreased or stayed the same since that time?"

"I suppose it's about the **same since then**. The reason I came in was that it **isn't getting any better**, you know."

"Yeah, I agree with you coming in. It can help if we can certainly find a reason for this pain. I'd like to gather some more information from you, then do a physical exam, and then we'll come up with a plan to approach this, ok?"

"Ok. Sounds fine."

"Have you had any other symptoms along with this? Such as fever or anything you can't explain?"

"Well, **no**, not really. I've been feeling **kind of run down lately** but nothing out of the ordinary."

"What do you mean 'run down?'"

"Well, I wouldn't mention this; I think its part of getting old. I've been feeling pretty tired lately. I've had a lot of **body aches** and seems like I can't go until the end of the day without pooping out. I get so tired that I need a **couple of naps** during the day. Like I said, I think it's my age."

Back pain "Red Flag" symptoms:
Fever
Weight loss
Loss of bowel/bladder control
Saddle anesthesia
Loss of sensory/motor control

Unprovoked back pain in the elderly should immediately raise your suspicions of malignancy.

Always treat the pain scale as the subjective assessment that it is. Some patients may minimize their score, whereas others may exaggerate.

"Well, age might have something to do with it, but there are a few other medical issues that might give you that feeling as well. Have you lost any weight at all?"

"**Yeah**, I've been losing weight for about a year now. Martha, my wife, died last year, and I started cooking for myself. I've gotten the hang of it; **I eat out a lot**, but I'm still losing some weight."

"How much weight have you lost in the past month, would you say?"

"Well, I don't keep track religiously, but I think about **10 pounds** over the **last month**."

"Do you think that's lack of appetite or not eating regularly or what?"

"Well, I **eat all the time**. I cook about one meal a day, usually breakfast, and then go out for another one. I **eat ok but just keep losing weight**. I don't know why, honestly."

"Ok. Have you had any other symptoms?"

"I think that's it."

"How about vision changes or lightheadedness?"

"My vision is the same—terrible. But my **glasses haven't changed**. I'm clear in the head, too."

"Ok. Any chest pain or trouble breathing?"

"**No**. I **smoked** for **40 years,** but since I quit 10 years ago, I've always said I can breathe easier."

"How about abdominal pain or nausea?"

"**None** of that."

"Any constipation or diarrhea?"

"A little **diarrhea** when I **eat fruit**. I avoid things like cherries and plums because of it. No problems otherwise."

"How about trouble urinating? Any trouble starting a stream?"

"**Yeah**, that's there, but it's been like that since I told my doctor and he gave me that medicine for it. He called it a **big prostate gland**."

"Ok. Did he mention benign prostatic hypertrophy or BPH? That's another term for a large prostate that isn't thought to have prostate cancer in it."

"Yeah, that sounds familiar; I'm taking tamsulosin for it."

"But you're still having a problem?"

"Yeah, well, I have **trouble starting to go**, like I have to put some pressure behind the pee. Then when I do go, it's a **dribble** sort of. **Not very much comes out**. Seems like I don't get it all out either, so it's not too long before I'm back in the bathroom."

"Ok. How long has this been going on?"

"Oh, probably about **5 or 6 years**. It's been slowly **getting worse**, though."

"Ok. Does it burn when you urinate?"

"**No**, no."

"Do you ever have any unusual discharge from your penis?"

> Don't ignore patients with minor complaints on review of systems. The unifying diagnosis may yet to be revealed.

"**No**, nothing."

"Have you seen the doctor for this since starting the medicine?"

"**No**, no. I've not mentioned it because I'm on that medicine. I see him about once every few months, and he did what he can do, so I haven't brought it up."

"Ok. Well, it's something I'd like to explore a little bit more with you today. Any other problems with urination?"

"**No**, that about covers it."

"Ok. Please tell me more about what other health problems you see the doctor about."

"Well, I have **high blood pressure**, I take medicine for that. I have **high cholesterol**, I take medicine for that. I have that **prostate problem**, we talked about that. I'm getting **cataracts,** and my doctor said when they get bad enough, I can have an operation for those. And I've also got **emphysema** from all that smoking. I'm on a breathing medicine for that. That's enough I think."

"Yeah, that's enough isn't it? Do you ever have trouble remembering all that medication?"

"**Nah**, I do ok."

"What are the names of all those medicines you're taking?"

"I have them here on my list. I'm taking **metoprolol**, **benazepril** for blood pressure. **Atorvastatin** for high cholesterol. **Tamsulosin**, like I mentioned for my prostate, and **tiotropium** inhaler for emphysema. I sometimes take **albuterol** if I need it but only really rarely. I've been known to take some **Tums** from time to time, too, for indigestion."

"Have you had a test called a colonoscopy in the last 5 to 10 years to look at your colon for cancer?"

"**Yeah**, boy do I remember that! It was about **4 years ago**. I remember that, and I don't want it again."

"Ok. Have you had any surgeries in your life?"

"Well, I **broke my left leg** in seven different places when I was in the Navy. I was in the war and had to jump ship. I hit a piece of debris when I hit the water. I had a few surgeries for that. It healed great, though, thanks to the docs. Then I had my **gallbladder out** when I was in the forest service, about 20 years ago now. I had a **hernia** here in my **groin** about 8 years ago. That's all my surgeries."

"Alright. I know you said you quit smoking. How much did you smoke when you did?"

"I smoked a **pack a day** for **40 years**. Quit when my doctor told me I was going to die from it. That was **ten years ago**."

"Have you had any trouble breathing or coughing lately?"

"No, I **cough in the morning** usually but I don't have problems with it."

"Do you ever cough up blood?"

Shyness or the desire to not "bother" the doctor with related health issues may be a barrier.

Patients on multiple medications often benefit from written medication lists. However, an updated and current list every time they see the physician is crucial to their care.

"**No**, never."

"Ok. Do you drink alcohol?"

"**No**, not anymore."

"Ok. Are there any diseases that have run in your family?"

"**No**. I've got three girls and they're all healthy with their families. My youngest just had twins. **My wife passed away about a year ago**. She had Parkinson's disease. It was better that way."

"Yeah, sometimes it is better when someone is suffering. Do you still feel sad or depressed because she's gone?"

"**Yeah**, of course. But that's the way it is. It was her time, and that disease wiped her out. It's better she's not suffering anymore, really."

"Do you ever feel like hurting yourself because you feel sad?"

"Oh, **no**, doc. I'd never do that."

> If a patient admits a major life stressor, screen for suicidal ideation.

Signpost for the Physical Exam

"Ok. I'd like to do a physical exam now, if you don't mind. Just let me **wash my hands.** First I'd like to listen to your lungs…"

Objective

Points for Every Exam:

- Wash hands.
- Comment on vital signs, even if normal.
- Tell the patient where you are going to examine and disrobe.
- Do not repeat painful maneuvers.

Physical Exam:

Perform a focused physical, by system, from the head down.

System	Exam elements	Findings in this patient
General	Note general appearance. Ill-appearing? Cachetic?	Cachetic-appearing with temporal wasting
Lungs	Auscultate the posterior and lateral lung fields. Make sure to listen to 6 points on the posterior lung fields.	Slight end expiratory wheeze heard. Mild rhonchi at lung bases bilaterally. No rales. Good breath sounds.
Abdomen	Observe for ecchymosis or skin changes. Listen for bowel sounds or bruit's. Palpate all 4 quadrants, perform Murphy's sign, and assess rebound tenderness over McBurney's point. Note any organomegaly.	Normal appearance. No ascites. No masses. BSs present, no bruit's. No ttp. Murphy's sign negative. No rebound tenderness. No hepatosplenomegaly.

Back	Observe for erythema, swelling, deformity, or spasm in the upright and sitting positions. Ask the patient to point to the maximum area of pain; avoid that area at first, then palpate it last. Note ischial spine relative height. Complete ROM maneuvers, including flexion, extension, lateral, and rotation, communicating with the patient to determine the most painful maneuvers or radiation of pain. Complete ipsilateral and contralateral leg raise testing.	The patient points to the approximate L3 level stating pain is midline and right-sided. Palpation of the spinous processes in the area produces exquisite tenderness. Palpation of the right praspinal area also produces tenderness. Flexion and extension are limited by pain. Rotational and lateral ROM is also limited by pain. Radiation of pain is reported with flexion and extension maneuvers. Negative leg raise testing.
Neurologic	Asses tactile sense of the lower extremities along with proprioception and sharp/dull testing. Perform deep tendon reflexes tests and motor strength testing. Observe gait including heel- and toe-walks.	Normal sensory and motor exams. Reflexes 2+ and symmetric. Sharp/dull testing normal. Heel- and toe-walks normal. Gait normal.

Continue to gather information as you do the physical exam. Comment aloud on any real or simulated abnormalities.

Example: *"I'm going to raise your whole leg up myself. Please tell me if you have pain in your back or if any pain radiates down your leg."*

Example: *"Please take a deep breath while I listen to your lungs."*

End of Case

End by explaining you have several ideas of what could be wrong and could cause these symptoms. Tell the patient the first two diagnoses on your differential list and the major tests you'd now like to perform.

Example: *"Ok, Mr. Shuman, the symptoms you're having in your back may likely be caused by a benign cause, such as muscle spasm or local inflammation. However, because you've been having this a while, and the pain goes down your leg, I'm concerned about one of the nerves in your back could be compressed. Nerve compression can sometimes happen from several different sources, including a slipped or bulging disc between the bones of the spine or arthritis and bone spurs in the area. Those are the most common causes; however, sometimes other things can compress the nerve, such as a rare occurrence like a cancerous tumor or a fracture of the back itself. The concerning aspect to your symptoms is also that you have that prostate problem that hasn't been checked on in a while. So today, I'd also like to do a prostate exam, which will involve a digital rectal exam, and get some blood work to evaluate you. This will give a better picture of any possible cancer that might be growing in the prostate gland, or elsewhere in the body. Prostate cancer is concerning since, when it travels to other parts of the body, it sometimes goes to the back. Like I said, however, its only one possibility but one we should definitely screen for.*

Another test I'll want to order on you today is a MRI scan of your back. This will check for the presence of a fracture or nerve compression. The MRI really allows us to look at the nerves exiting the back in a more detailed manner. I'll just need to step out for a few minutes to arrange these with my nurse.

I know this is a lot to absorb all at once. Remember, right now, we are just trying to find out why you might have this pain. Do you have any questions or is there any other aspect of your health care we haven't already discussed? Ok then, thank you."

PATIENT NOTE

History: Include significant positives and negatives from history of present illness, past medical history, review of system(s), social history, and family history.

HPI: 73 y/o male with lumbar back pain x 3 weeks. Pain reported as spontaneous without provocation and accompanied by midline tenderness and radiation down the right lower extremity. Pain is described as 4/10 intensity noticeable at night. ROS positive for recent fatigue and weight loss. No loss of bowel or bladder function although concurrent symptomatic BPH also noted in history. BPH has not been followed up recently and symptoms of weakened urinary stream and subjective urinary retention are worsening. He denies fever, nausea, decreased PO intake, changes in vision, or mental status change.

PMH: Hypertension—treated; hyperlipidemia—treated; emphysema—treated; GERD—treated, BPH—treated.

PSH: Fractured leg—historic; hernia—historic; cholecystectomy—historic.

Tobacco: 40 pack-years. Quit x 10 yrs.

EtOH: Denies.

Social history: Wife deceased x 1 year. Pt admits to feelings of bereavement but denies SI/HI.

Meds: metoprolol, benazepril, tiotropium inhaled, albuterol inhaled, tamsulosin, occasional antacids.

Physical Examination: Indicate only pertinent positive and negative findings related to the patient's chief complaint.

VVS Stable.

Lungs: Good breath sounds. Slight end expiratory wheeze. Mild rhonchi at lung bases bilaterally. No rales.

Abdomen: Normal appearance. No masses. BSs present, no bruit. No ttp. Murphy's sign negative. No rebound tenderness.

Back: TTP at L3 level over spinous process and right paraspinal area. Flexion and extension limited by pain. Rotational and lateral ROM also limited by pain. Radiation of pain down right leg in dermatomal distribution reported with flexion and extension maneuvers. Negative straight leg raise testing.

Neuro: Normal tactile sense, proprioception, sharp/dull normal. Motor strength 5/5 bilaterally. Reflexes 2+ and symmetric. Heel- and toe-walks normal. Gait normal.

Differential Diagnosis: In order of likelihood (with 1 being the most likely), list up to 5 potential or possible diagnoses for this patient's presentation (in many cases, fewer than 5 diagnoses are likely)	Diagnostic Work-up: List immediate plans (up to 5) for further diagnostic work-up
1. Metastatic cancer to the lumbar spine	1. Prostate/digital rectal exam
2. Pathologic fracture	2. PSA
3. Degenerative joint disease and spondylosis	3. MRI back
4. Intervertebral disc herniation or rupture	4. Electrolytes, renal function, liver enzyme panel, alkaline phosphatase.
5. Osteoporotic fracture	5. CBC with manual differential

25 Shoulder Pain

1. Opening Scenario

Michael McKinney, a 34-year-old male, comes to the clinic complaining of right-sided shoulder pain.

2. Vital Signs

BP: 138/88 mmHg

Temp: 98.4° F (36.9° C)

HR: 60/minute, regular

RR: 16/minute

3. Examinee Tasks

1. Obtain a focused history.

2. Perform a relevant physical examination. (Do not perform breast, pelvic/genital, or rectal examination.)

3. Discuss your initial diagnostic impression and your work-up plan.

4. After leaving the room, complete your patient note on the given form.

Are the Vital Signs Stable?

Subjective

Knock; enter. Introduce yourself, and place the first signpost.

"Hello, Mr. McKinney, I'm Dr. Nelson. I understand you've had some shoulder pain lately. Please tell me more about it."

"Hi doctor. Yeah, I've been having **shoulder pain** for about **2 months now**. It hurts like crazy when I'm trying to **sleep** or **working out**. I don't really know what caused it. It's right here [pointing to the anterior right shoulder]."

"Ok. Let me ask some questions of you first, then I'd like to examine you fully. I know you said you don't know what caused it, but do you remember a first time you injured it, such as a direct blow or a strain?"

"Well, it just came on during **the softball season**. I used to play on a team and was the **first baseman**. I'm right-handed, so this is my **throwing**

> Provoking factors for shoulder pain are especially important.

shoulder, but it only really started at the **end of the season**. There really **wasn't any specific time** I threw it out or anything; it just started hurting then. I seem to have the worst pain when I'm in bed at night. I roll over or something and it hurts and I have to find another position."

"I can imagine how uncomfortable that might be. Does anything else bring on the pain?"

"Well, like I said, **weight-lifting** does. I go to the gym about every other day. It hurts when I do the **bench press** or pretty much do **anything really strenuous** with that shoulder. When I do overhead stuff it hurts the most. I mean, I only really do my upper body every other time I go to the gym. Otherwise I'm working my legs and abs, you know."

"Has the area ever gotten red or swollen?"

"**Nah**, it just hurts. I can't tell from looking at it."

"Ok. Have you done anything for the pain such as taken medication?"

"I took a couple **naproxen** the **other day**. It helped a little, but I don't want to be on that stuff very long. I don't take it all the time. I took some **ibuprofen** about **2 weeks** ago, but that didn't help. That's why I tried the naproxen this time."

"How about a hot or cold pack?"

"**No**, never done that. Sometimes I go to the sauna, but that doesn't do anything."

"Alright. Does the pain radiate anywhere or stay in that spot?"

"It just **stays there** mainly. You know, it's just this one spot but kind of the front region [pointing to the right anterior shoulder region]."

"How about the quality of the pain—does it feel sharp or dull?"

"It's kind of a **sharp**. I don't have it all the time. For example, it isn't hurting when I'm sitting here talking to you. Just **certain movements**."

"On a scale of 0 to 10, 10 being the worst pain imaginable, where would you rate this pain at its worst?"

"At its **worst**? Probably a **7** or so. That's when it's really bugging me. Like I said, it **doesn't hurt all the time**."

"Sure. Is there a time of day it hurts worse?"

"Well, **not really**. I'm more active toward the end of the day, so probably then."

"Has your shoulder felt unstable, as if it will easily pop out of place?"

"**No**, it doesn't feel like that."

"Have you ever dislocated that shoulder?"

"Nope."

"Has it ever locked up so you can't move it?"

"**No**."

"Are you having any tingling sensation or numbness in that arm or hand?"

"**No**, no problems with that."

"Have you had any chest pain or trouble breathing lately?"

"**No**, not at all."

"Any chest congestion or cough?"

"**Nope**."

"How about any pain in your abdomen?"

"**No**, none of that."

"Have you had any other problems with your joints or muscles?"

"Well, I'm a pretty athletic guy so I've **broken my thumb** once and **sprained both ankles** many times. Nothing out of the ordinary, though. I'm also **a police officer,** and 2 years ago I was **shot in the right leg**. It was just in the muscle, though, kind of grazed me, you know? I recovered pretty well. They said I was lucky."

"Sounds like you were—that's a tough line of work. Ok. How about other problems in your past medical history? Anything you've seen the doctor for, or stayed in the hospital for other than what you mentioned?"

"Um, well, I have seen the doctor for **erectile dysfunction**. It happens sometimes. He gave me medicine called **vardenafil**. I only take it occasionally. I haven't stayed the night in the hospital ever."

"Ok. How about surgeries, other than that gunshot wound?"

"Yeah, I had my **tonsils out** when I was 12 years old. Otherwise, nothing."

"I have the vardenifil, occasional naproxen, and ibuprofen. Are you on any other medicines?"

"I have **eczema** on my elbows. I put a steroid on it when it gets bad. That's only when I need it, though."

"Ok. Is that only a topical medicine?"

"**Yeah**. It's been a few months since I had to put any on."

"Alright. Do you smoke or use tobacco?"

"**No**, no. I'm pretty healthy."

"Do you drink alcohol at all?"

"I drink occasionally. Maybe a beer with dinner every now and again. Maybe once a week."

"Ok. Any other drugs?"

"**No,** never."

How about dietary supplements?"

"**No**, I used to but just haven't kept up with it."

"Ok. Has there been any major diseases in your family at all?"

"**No**, both parents are good. I have two sisters, both are fine."

It's important to ask about abdomen and chest pain when evaluating shoulder problems because some pathology in those systems may produce referred shoulder pain.

Signpost for the Physical Exam

"Ok. I'd like to do a physical exam now, if you don't mind. Just let me wash my hands. It looks like your **vital signs are normal,** so please remove your shirt so I can take a look at your shoulders…"

Objective

Points for Every Exam:

- Wash hands.
- Comment on vital signs, even if normal.
- Tell the patient where you are going to examine and disrobe.
- Do not repeat painful maneuvers.

Physical Exam:

Perform a focused physical, by system, from the head down.

System	Exam elements	Findings in this patient
Neurologic	Assess tactile sense of both upper extremities. Test deep tendon reflexes and muscle strength.	Normal tactile sensation, DTRs, and 5/5 motor strength
Musculoskeletal	Observe both shoulders for symmetry or obvious differences. Ask the patient where his pain is and palpate the region as well as other landmarks of shoulder. Concentrate on the right and start with passive ROM followed by active. Assess flexion, extension, abduction/adduction, and external/internal rotation. Conduct relative strength testing the move onto special tests: cross-arm test, Neer's test, Hawkin's test, isometric supraspinatus and infraspinatus tests, "empty-can" tests, passive arc maneuver, Speed's test, and Yergason's test.	Symmetric appearance. Mild tenderness to palpation over anterior glenohumoral region. No tenderness over coracoid process or biceps tendon. Full ROM. No sulcus sign. Neer's test and "empty-can" test positive for impingement. Cross-arm test mildly positive. Suprasinatus isometric testing positive. Internal and external strength normal, Speed's test negative, Yergason's test negative. No apprehension during maneuvers.

Continue to gather information as you do the physical exam. Comment aloud on any real or simulated abnormalities.

Example: *"Does this maneuver cause an increase in pain?"*

Example: *"Can you show me what makes this pain worse?"*

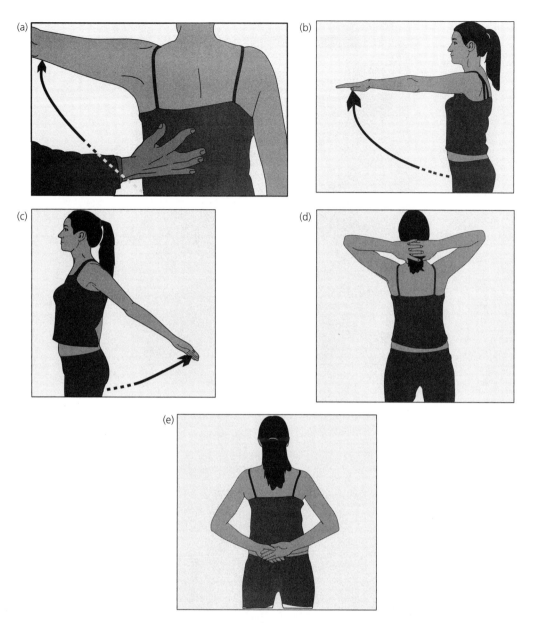

FIGURE 25.1 Assessing shoulder movements. (a) Abduction, (b) Flexion, (c) Extension, (d) External rotation, (e) Internal rotation.

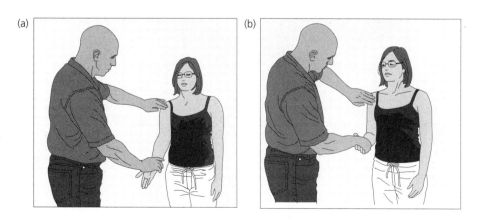

FIGURE 25.2 Biceps tendon tests. (a) Speed's test. (b) Yergason's test.

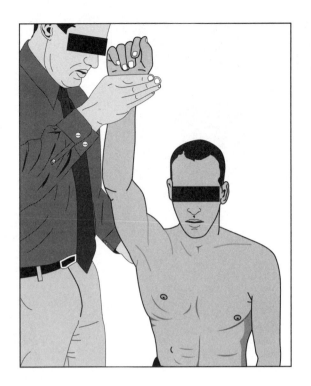

FIGURE 25.3 Neer test.

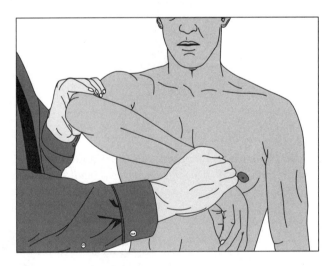

FIGURE 25.4 Hawkins test.

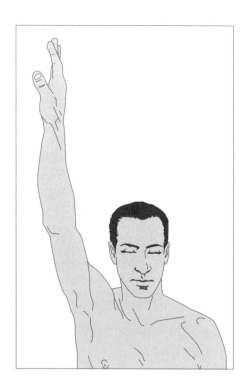

FIGURE 25.5 Painful arc test.

End of Case

End by explaining you have several ideas of what could be wrong and could cause these symptoms. Tell the patient the first two diagnoses on your differential list and the major tests you'd now like to perform.

Example: *"Mr. McKinney, there are a few possibilities that might be causing your pain based on what you've told me and my physical exam, I think it could be caused by direct inflammation to the tendons that make up what's called the rotator cuff. The rotator cuff is a set of muscles and tendons that hold the shoulder joint together and provide the muscle power to move it. These tendons may be injured by straining or partial tearing as is likely in your case. The sheaths around the tendon often get inflamed because of this. This inflammation causes what's called 'impingement,' which is the trapping of inflamed tendon sheaths between two opposing bones in the shoulder. This occurs when the tendon itself is torn or inflamed or the sheath around it gets inflamed, causing it to enlarge slightly. Because the shoulder has so much going on in a small space, these inflamed and enlarged tendons sometimes get caught between areas of bone, which causes pain. Another possibility is that there's a small tear in the cup that holds the ball of the shoulder in place. The tear can be an irritation that occurs with certain types of movement causing your pain. Although I think this is less likely, I'd like to start you on some therapy here in the clinic and see you again in follow up in a few weeks to assess how it's going. The therapy will be with a constant dose of the medicine you've tried, Naprosyn. This works to reduce the inflammation in that area and calm the irritation. This medicine should be taken constantly over the next few weeks and I'm also going to advise you not to strain that shoulder in this time. I recommend no weight-lifting or any sports that may cause strain of that area. The more it's strained, the more inflammation can occur, which starts the cycle over again. There are other therapies that might be of use to employ if this trial of therapy isn't successful. However, starting this medicine and having you follow-up is the best course of action right now. If we have to, we may need to go to the next step at your next appointment. That includes possibly injecting that shoulder with a steroid or obtaining a diagnostic study such as an MRI. I hope, however, we can take care of this without those next steps. Do you have any questions about your diagnosis or your treatment course?*

Is there any other aspect of your health care we haven't already discussed? Ok then, thank you."

PATIENT NOTE

History: Include significant positives and negatives from history of present illness, past medical history, review of system(s), social history, and family history.

HPI: 34 y/o male with right anterior shoulder pain x 2 months. Original injury in conjunction with sports, baseball-throwing, although no specific event/trauma. Pain described as sharp, nonradiating, 7/10 at worst, although 0/10 when not provoked. Pain exacerbated by weight-lifting, overhead strain, and is worse at night. Denies dislocation or instability. Denies locking or radiating neurologic symptoms. Not relieved by intermittent naproxen or ibuprofen.

ROS: No chest pain, abdominal pain, or respiratory complaints. Otherwise noncontributory.

PMH: Fractured left thumb. Multiple ankle sprains. Gunshot wound, right thigh. Eczema. Erectile dysfunction.

PSH: Tonsillectomy; repair gunshot wound to right thigh.

Meds: Inconsistent use of naproxen and ibuprofen. Occasional vardenifil. Intermittent topical steroids.

Tobacco: Denies.

Alcohol use: Socially.

FamH: Noncontributory.

Physical Examination: Indicate only pertinent positive and negative findings related to the patient's chief complaint.

VS Stable, normal.

Neuro: Upper extremities: Strength 5/5 throughout, tactile sensation normal, Reflexes 2+ bilaterally.

MS: Symmetric appearance, no erythema/deformity. Mild ttp over anterior glenohumoral region. Full ROM. No sulcus sign. Neer's test and "empty can" test positive. Cross arm test mildly positive. Suprasinatus isometric testing positive. Internal/external strength normal, Speed's test negative, Yergason's test negative. No apprehension during maneuvers.

Differential Diagnosis: In order of likelihood (with 1 being the most likely), list up to 5 potential or possible diagnoses for this patient's presentation (in many cases, fewer than 5 diagnoses are likely)	Diagnostic Work-up: List immediate plans (up to 5) for further diagnostic work-up
1. Rotator cuff tendonopathy	1.
2. Impingement syndrome	2.
3. Tear of the glenoid labrum (SLAP lesion)	3.
4. Osteoarthritis	4.
5. Biceps tendonitis	5.

---

1. Opening Scenario

Wendy Nickels, a 43-year-old female, presents to the emergency department for evaluation of pain in the right leg lasting 24 hours.

2. Vital Signs

BP:	142/87 mmHg
Temp:	98.6° F (37.0° C)
HR:	70/minute, regular
RR:	12/minute
Pulse oximetry:	98% on room air

3. Examinee Tasks

1. Obtain a focused history.
2. Perform a relevant physical examination. (Do not perform breast, pelvic/genital, or rectal examination.)
3. Discuss your initial diagnostic impression and your work-up plan.
4. After leaving the room, complete your patient note on the given form.

Are the Vital Signs Stable?

Subjective

Knock; enter. Introduce yourself, and place the first signpost.

"Hello Ms. Nickels, I'm Dr. Torrado. I understand you've been having some pain in your leg? Can you tell me about that?"

"Hello, doctor. Yes, this **pain started yesterday**. I was **driving** home from my father's house and noticed it when I got out of the car. My **calf** was sort of sore, and it's strange, but it **felt hot,** you know. Now, I had just been helping with his **gardening** over the weekend and part of that was mowing down these tall weeds on his property. Well, there were all sorts of things in those weeds so, well, maybe I got into something. Anyway, so the next day, this morning, I got up, and it was **red and hot and more painful**. I figured I'd just tough it out and go to work. I work at a law office and couldn't get away all day to come in but it was really hurting. Maybe I was just obsessive. Anyway, so after work my regular doctor was closed so I thought I should come here rather than let it go anymore."

"Alright. Did you have any symptoms before mowing the weeds?"

"**Nope**, and it was more like after I got out of the car from driving home."

"How long of a drive was it?"

"It's **5 hours**. He lives in San Andreas."

"How about your other leg or other parts of your body? Has anywhere else been sore?"

"**No**, it's just that leg, here on the **back** [rubbing the posterior right calf]."

"Ok. Other than the redness, has there been any oozing or scaling?"

"No, none of that. Just **hot and sore and red** throughout today. I think it's **swollen**, too."

"Does the pain radiate anywhere?"

"**No,** it stays in that spot."

"Does anything make the pain worse, such as walking or standing on your tip-toes?"

"Well, **yeah**. It hurts to really **stretch** it or **walk** vigorously or **stand on my toes**. The **skin feels tight**, you know?"

"I can imagine it's uncomfortable. Have you taken anything for the pain? Any medication?"

> Throughout the interview, use empathetic statements toward symptoms.

"I took some **ibuprofen** this morning. That helped a little, maybe. But not much."

"Do you feel like it's gotten worse over the day?"

"**Yeah**, I do. Maybe it's because I've been so active on it, but it hurts bad enough to come into the ER. And I never come into the hospital."

"On a scale of 0 to 10, 10 being the worst pain imaginable, where would you place this pain at its worst?"

"I'd say an **8**. It hurts the most when I **walk** though."

"Have you had a fever or felt hot in the last day?"

"**No**, not really."

"How about any breathing problems, like pain when breathing or breathing fast?"

"**No**, I would have come in right away if I had that."

"Anything else, like numbness or tingling in that foot or leg?"

"Um, **no**, the foot feels about the same."

"Have you felt lightheaded or dizzy during this illness?"

"**No**, not at all."

"Has a similar episode ever happened to you before?"

> Acknowledge the patient's diagnostic suggestions. It can give important clues to the ultimate diagnosis.

"**No never**, this is the first time. I thought it might be poison ivy but a friend of mine told me she didn't think so."

"That may be one possibility. Have you gotten any rashes before? Even ones that don't look like this?"

"I got a **rash** to a medication called **amoxicillin** once when I was in college. It made me break out on my stomach and chest. Nothing else though."

"That brings up another good point—are you allergic to anything?"

"Nothing other than **amoxicillin**."

"Are you on any medications now?"

"I'm on my **birth control patch**. It's called Ortho Evra. I put it on my arm once a week. I'm also on **Paxil** for **anxiety**."

"Ok. How long have you taken these?"

"About **2 years** for the patch. Maybe **6 months** for the Paxil."

"Alright. Do you smoke?"

"I **used to**. I smoked for 20 years. Quit 2 years ago when I got on birth control. My doctor helped me get off of it. None of that since I quit."

"How much every day did you smoke?"

"About a **pack a day** for most of that time. At the end I weaned down slowly with those nicotine patches."

"Great. You know, it's a great thing that you stopped smoking. It's something many people try to do for a long time. Well done. Let me ask about alcohol— any of that?"

> Take every effort to encourage quitting smoking. Reaffirmation by a physician does contribute to success rates.

"I drink maybe a **glass of wine or beer** on the **weekend or at parties**. I mean, it's not much more than 2 or 3 nights per week."

"Have you ever tried to cut down?"

"**No**, never felt I had to."

"Have you ever felt guilty because of your drinking?"

"**No**."

"Have you ever had an 'eye opener,' or a drink in the morning?"

"Oh **no**."

"Have you ever felt annoyed by someone else talking about your alcohol consumption?"

"**No**."

> When moderate alcohol exposure is found, ask the four CAGE questions.
> Cut down?
> Annoyed?
> Guilty?
> Eye opener?

"Alright, have you ever taken any other drugs for pleasure?"

"Well, I tried **cocaine** once when I was in **grad school**. I hated it, and it didn't feel good. Never again. Nothing else."

"Alright. Have you ever been to the doctor for anything serious in your life? Anything you've stayed in the hospital for?"

"**No**, I've just seen my doctor for that anxiety thing and for my yearly exam."

"Have you ever been pregnant?"

"**No**, I've never felt I wanted kids."

"Have you ever had an abnormal pap smear or mammogram?"

"**No**, never."

"Have you ever had problems bleeding or clotting your blood?"

"**Nope**."

"Let me ask about your family a little. Has anyone in your family ever had a major disease?"

"My mom had **lung cancer** 4 years ago now. It was the kind that she needed to be on chemotherapy and have surgery. She smoked all her life. She's doing alright now. My dad died in a housefire years ago. He was a firefighter. My two younger brothers are both healthy. Actually, one is on medicine for high **blood pressure,** now that I think of it."

Signpost for the Physical Exam

"Ok. I'd like to do a physical exam now, if you don't mind. Just let me **wash my hands.** Please let me ask you to pull up your gown so I may first look at that leg…"

Objective

Points for Every Exam:

- Wash hands.
- Comment on vital signs, even if normal.
- Tell the patient where you are going to examine and disrobe.
- Do not repeat painful maneuvers.

Physical Exam:

Perform a focused physical, by system, from the head down.

System	Exam elements	Findings in this patient
Lungs	Auscultate the posterior and lateral lung fields. Make sure to listen to 6 points on the posterior lung fields and 1 on each lateral lung field.	Clear to auscultation bilaterally Normal breath sounds, no wheezes, rhonichi, or rales.
Heart	Listen for heart sounds in at least 4 different auscultation points. Feel for the point of maximal impulse (PMI). While auscultatiing the heart, palpate the radial pulses. Check the capillary refill time.	RRR no murmurs/rubs/gallops. Peripheral pulses 2+ bilaterally. Cap refill <2 secs. BP normal.
Lower extremities	Observe and compare the unaffected and affected lower extremities. Start with inspection of the general appearance, then palpate distal pulses, feel for warmth, assess tenderness, and assess ROM of the knee and ankle joints. Make sure to examine with a light and measure each calf diameter with measuring tape. Comment on any fluctuance or induration you feel. Check for popliteal, femoral, or inguinal lymphadenopathy. Check Homan's sign. Comment on palpable cords you feel.	Erythema noted on exam. No skin break or scaling of skin. Tenderness noted to the touch. No fluctuance noted. Mild induration of entire right calf region. Mild swelling noted, with 1 cm difference in calf circumferences. Erythema approx 3x5 cm and elliptical in shape. Pulses, including popliteal, posterior tibial, and dorsalis pedis, all normal. No palpable lymphadenopathy. Mildly positive Homan's sign. Neg palpable cords.

Continue to gather information as you do the physical exam. Comment aloud on any real or simulated abnormalities.

Example: *"Do you have much pain when I move your foot like this* [during dorsiflexion of the foot in checking Homan's sign].*"*

Example: *"Please take a deep breath while I listen to your back."*

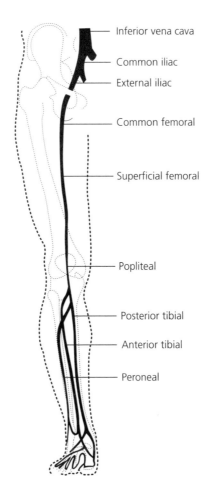

Inferior vena cava
Common iliac
External iliac
Common femoral
Superficial femoral
Popliteal
Posterior tibial
Anterior tibial
Peroneal

FIGURE 26.1 Location of deep vein thromboses.

End of Case

End by explaining you have several ideas of what could be wrong and could cause these symptoms. Tell the patient the first two diagnoses on your differential list and the major tests you'd now like to perform.

Example: *"Ms. Nickels, I think your symptoms may result from several different problems. The most serious is that you may have a blood clot in one of the deep veins of your leg. That may be causing your symptoms and by itself isn't absolutely concerning. However, the big problem with a blood clot there is that a small piece may break off and travel in your bloodstream to your lung, where it can get lodged. That's called a pulmonary embolism and is a much more serious condition. I can test for a blood clot in your leg with a special machine that uses sound waves to look at blood flow through the veins. I'll also want to get some blood work for this possibility. Another possibility is that you have an infection of the skin in that part of your leg. That type of infection is most commonly caused by a skin bacteria somehow getting under and into the skin and growing. That may have happened during the gardening you mentioned. I'd also like to evaluate that with some blood work. There are several other possibilities that I'll also be looking for with these tests. To get you started, however, I'd like to step out and place the orders. It will only take a few minutes.*

Is there any other aspect of your health care we haven't already discussed? Ok then, thank you."

PATIENT NOTE

History: Include significant positives and negatives from history of present illness, past medical history, review of system(s), social history, and family history.

HPI: 43 y/o female c/o right calf pain accompanied by local swelling, redness, and warmth x 24 hours. She reports onset of symptoms after long car trip but also states recent exposure to tall grass while gardening. Pain worsened by walking and plantar flexing foot. Symptoms gradually worsening since onset. Denies fever, tachypnea, pleurisy, or chest pain. This is her first episode of similar pain and is 8/10. OTC strength ibuprofen showed mild relief of symptoms.

PMH: G0P0. Anxiety—treated.

PSH: None.

Tobacco: 20 pack-years. Quit smoking cigarettes x 2 years.

EtOH: Occasional. CAGE questions negative.

Drugs: Historic use of cocaine x 1.

Meds: Ortho Evra patch. Paxil. Recent ibuprofen.

FamH: Mother—lung cancer; father—deceased, trauma; brother—hypertension.

Physical Examination: Indicate only pertinent positive and negative findings related to the patient's chief complaint.

VS Stable.

Heart: RRR no murmurs/rubs/gallops. Clear S1/S2. Pulses 2+ throughout. Cap refill <2 secs.

Lungs: Clear to auscultation bilaterally. No wheezes/rubs/rhonchi.

Lower extremities: Right posterior lower ext: + erythema without defined borders—approx 3x5 cm, elliptical. No skin break noted. Neg fluctuance. Mild generalized induration. Mildly positive Homan's sign. Difference in calf circumference 1 cm. 2+ pulses in popliteal, post-tibial, and dorsalis pedis. No palpable cords.

Differential Diagnosis: In order of likelihood (with 1 being the most likely), list up to 5 potential or possible diagnoses for this patient's presentation (in many cases, fewer than 5 diagnoses are likely)	Diagnostic Work-up: List immediate plans (up to 5) for further diagnostic work-up
1. Deep Vein Thrombosis (DVT)	1. Doppler compression ultrasound
2. Cellulitis	2. CBC with differential
3. Contact dermatitis	3. D-dimer
4. superficial thrombophlebitis	4.
5. Envenomation	5.

27 Fatigue and Bruising

1. Opening Scenario

John Clarkson, a 62-year-old male, presents with complaints of fatigue and bruising.

2. Vital Signs

BP: 140/85 mmHg

Temp: 98.4° F (36.9° C)

HR: 66/minute, regular

RR: 12/minute

3. Examinee Tasks

1. Obtain a focused history.

2. Perform a relevant physical examination. (Do not perform breast, pelvic/genital, or rectal examination.)

3. Discuss your initial diagnostic impression and your work-up plan.

4. After leaving the room, complete your patient note on the given form.

Are the Vital Signs Stable?

Subjective

Knock, enter. Introduce yourself, and place the first signpost.

"Hi Mr. Clarkson, I'm Dr. Wanik. I understand you've been having some fatigue and skin bruising. Please tell me what's going on with this."

"Yeah, doc, I'm just tired. I've been **really beat** for the last **3 weeks** or so. I just can't tell you what it is, but I can hardly keep my eyes open. I'm a tugboat driver on the river. I usually work some pretty crazy hours, but this is **more than that**. I haven't fallen asleep on the job or anything, but I'm really, really beat all the time. It ain't like me, ya know?"

"Have you changed the time you work at all? That is, do you work night and day shifts?"

When a patient is doing a job that may endanger himself or others, symptoms that alter work performance may be critical.

"**No**, I work in the daytime, but it's pretty much from sun-up to sun-down. I've done that for 19 years, though. It's more like I feel like my bones and body just ache. I'm sleepy, too, but it's more like a constant fatigue, you know?"

"I'll bet that's tough when you're doing something that requires so much concentration. Did this just start 3 weeks ago, or have you ever had this feeling before?"

"Well, I've been tired before, sure, but this has really increased the last 3 weeks. I've **never** really had this before."

"Have you had any recent illnesses like a cold or flu?"

"**No**, not really. I'm always out in the weather, but I haven't been sick lately."

"What are your hours of sleep at night?"

"About…from maybe 11 o'clock to about 6:00 in the morning. That's like clockwork."

"Any trouble sleeping at all?"

"Nah, like I say, I sleep on a schedule and my body's just gotten used to it. I don't even need an alarm anymore. That's what 19 years on the job will do for you."

"I can imagine. Please tell me about this skin bruising you told my nurse about."

"Well, that's another thing. I've got these **big bruises**. Look at these [pulling up his sleeves]. It's on my arms and my hip. I bump things all the time, but it hasn't ever caused these. I've always got a cut or bruise somewhere, but these are huge and I don't even remember hitting anything bad enough to do it."

"When did these start appearing?"

"Well, I guess the **last few weeks**. This one here [pointing to his right hip] has been there for at least 2 weeks."

"Ok. I'll take a look at you everywhere in a few minutes. I can sure see them on your arms, though. Have you cut or torn your skin recently? Enough to bleed?"

"I do that all the time on accident. A fish hook or something. I did it the other day."

"Did it bleed for a long time?"

"Now that you mention it, yeah, it did. It bled for a while, and I had to get a second rag until it stopped. That is weird, now that you mention it."

"How about anything else going on? Anything else such as fever or sweating at night?

"**No**, I haven't had a fever. I **don't** really sweat much at night."

"Have you had any headaches or pain anywhere?"

"**No**, I rarely get headaches. As far as pain, it's just those aches in my body."

"Do those aches center around your joints or your muscles, or are they all over and hard to point to one place?"

"Well, it **hurts all over**. It's not really isolated anywhere. I'd say it's all over my muscles. My bones feel like they hurt, too, but it's all over. Kind of feels like when you get the flu and you have that really tired feeling. Yeah, it feels like that."

"How about eating—do you have an appetite?"

"Well, I might be eating a little less now. I guess I haven't wanted too much food but I can't tell you why, I'm just **not hungry**."

"Have you lost weight recently?"

"Actually, **I have**. I checked my weight last night and I'm usually about **250** or so; I've gone down to **239**. I was surprised; I haven't tried to do it. It just happened."

"Ok. Do you ever feel faint or like you might pass out?"

"**No**, no. That's not a problem."

"Do you ever have a change in your vision?"

"**No**, I'd notice that right away."

"Ok. Have you ever seen the doctor for anything in your life? Especially anything you stayed the night in the hospital for?"

"**Yeah**, I had a **blood clot in my lungs** 3 months ago. I felt just horrible and was coughing up blood and the whole bit. I eventually went in, and he said a clot **came from my leg** and got stuck in my lung. He put me on this medicine that's real important for me to take, so I do, every day."

"Ok. Only 3 months ago, huh? Do you remember the medicine you're on for that?"

"**No**, I can't remember the name. I don't remember."

"Would it be Warfarin?"

"That **sounds familiar**, **yeah**, I think so."

"Did the doctor adjust the dosage based on your blood work?"

"**Yeah,** he did."

"Ok. Are you taking that medicine as he directed?"

"**Yup**, every day."

"Are you on any other medicines?"

"I hate pills. I swallow an **aspirin** every day, too. I take **ibuprofen** every now and again for this or that."

"Have you taken the ibuprofen lately?"

"**No**, I thought the aspirin was the same thing. Isn't it?"

"Not exactly. It works the same way, but often aspirin is typically used to thin the blood, whereas ibuprofen is preferred for aches and pains.

Are you having trouble breathing lately as well?"

"**No**, all that went away after I went to the hospital for a while. I pay close attention to that now, and I don't have anything like it."

"How about breathing fast or trouble breathing?"

"**No**, breathing is fine."

"Do you now or have you ever smoked?"

"I smoked a **pack a day for 40 years**. Since this clot, I've cut back to about half a pack per day. I know it's bad for me, but it's something I've done for 40 years—kind of hard to quit altogether like the doc in the hospital told me."

"Would you like help with quitting?"

"Nah, I like it. Besides, it's my only vice anymore."

"Well, ok. Do you drink alcohol at all?"

"I **don't** have time. I'm working all the time, and by the time I get home, I'm just not interested."

Always decide if weight loss in a specific time is within normal variation. In men, this can be as much as 2–3 lbs in a few days.

Patients may neglect to admit major health events. This is why obtaining a past medical history on every patient is important.

It's very important to note if a medication name is only recognized and not named by the patient. That medication can never be assumed to be correct, and verification after immediate management is needed.

"How about any other drugs?"

"**No**, no. Not for me."

"Other than that blood clot, have you had any other trips to the doctor?"

"I had a **broken arm** about **5 years ago**. My tug was swept into a bridge piling. Broke my arm in the crash. That's all."

"Alright. How about any surgeries?"

"I had my **appendix** out when I was a **teenager**. Nothing else though."

"Ok. Are you married?"

"Nope, **divorced**. I've got three boys. All of them are in college, that's why I work so hard."

"Ok. How about any major diseases in your family, especially anything similar to this?"

"**No**, my **parents are both dead**. Mom from **smoking** at age **86** and dad from a **heart attack** at **76**. My **brother** in Philadelphia has **diabetes**. Nothing else, though."

Signpost for the Physical Exam

"Ok. I'd like to do a physical exam now, if you don't mind. Just let me wash my hands. It looks like your **vital signs are normal.** I'd like to first listen to your heart…

Objective

Points for Every Exam:

- Wash hands.
- Comment on vital signs, even if normal.
- Tell the patient where you are going to examine and disrobe.
- Do not repeat painful maneuvers.

Physical Exam:

Perform a focused physical, by system, from the head down.

System	Exam elements	Findings in this patient
Lymph nodes	Check the lymph node chains in the anterior/posterior cervical neck, axillary, supraclavicular, inguinal, femoral, and popliteal locations.	Moderate diffuse lymphadenopathy
Lung	Listen to 6 different areas of posterior lung fields.	Clear to auscultation bilaterally
Heart	Listen to 4 different areas on the anterior chest.	Regular, rate, and rhythm. No murmurs, rubs, or gallups heard.
Abdomen	Listen for bowel sounds and bruit's. Palpate in all 4 quadrants, noting any abnormalities aloud. Check Murphy's sign and rebound tenderness over McBurney's point. Percuss out the limits of the liver. Palpate for the spleen.	Bowel sounds normal. Murphy's sign negative. No rebound tenderness. No hepatomegally. Positive splenomegally with displaced spleen tip noted.
Skin	Check all parts of the skin, uncovering them sequentially as you go. Check arms, hands, legs, feet, abdomen, back, neck, and, lastly, groin, genitals, and hips. Note blanchability of lesions and if swelling is also present.	Large macular ecchymosis on arms and on anterior shins. Right hip with large ecchymosis.

Continue to gather information as you do the physical exam. Comment aloud on any real or simulated abnormalities.

Example: *"Are these bruises tender when I touch them?"*

Example: *"Have you noticed these lumps under your skin?"*

End of Case

End by explaining you have several ideas of what could be wrong and could cause these symptoms. Tell the patient the first two diagnoses on your differential list and the major tests you'd now like to perform.

Example: *"Mr. Clarkson, I can't tell exactly what is going on to produce your symptoms we talked about today. But there are a few things I'd like to take some tests for, and we can further figure it out. First, it might be that medicine you're on. That's one that can make you bruise easily, although it shouldn't cause the fatigue and weight that loss you've had. I can check a blood test to see if that's the problem. Another disease this might be is a rare cancer called leukemia. That's a type of cancer that forms in the blood and affects different areas of your body. In your case, I would be thinking of a specific type, but it's really much too early to tell. And this disease is very rare overall and only a small possibility in you. I'll be able to tell a little better with some blood work. If the results of the blood work suggest this might be a strong possibility, we would have to get some further testing— namely, a biopsy of your bone or lymph nodes—to tell for sure. So keep in mind, the blood work won't be able to say for sure one way or another. Also, this is only one unlikely possibility that is going on here. As far as some other possibilities, there are a few, and I'll also be running some lab work for them. For those, we'll need blood from a simple needle stick in your arm. I'd like to step out and arrange this with my nurse if you don't mind.*
Is there any other aspect of your health care we haven't already discussed? Ok then, thank you."

PATIENT NOTE

History: Include significant positives and negatives from history of present illness, past medical history, review of system(s), social history, and family history.

HPI: 62 y/o male c/o fatigue, weight loss, and easy bruising x 3 wks. He states fatigue involves tiredness and body aches similar to "flu-like symptoms." Weight loss unintentional and a/w mildly decreased appetite. Bruising reported from minor trauma and is out of proportion of injuries. No headache, fever, night sweats, or other constitutional symptoms. Prolonged bleeding to minor trauma also reported but controllable.

PMH: Pulmonary embolism a/w DVT—3 months ago. Fractured arm.

PSH: Appendectomy.

Tobacco: ½ pack per day. 40 pack-years.

Alcohol use: Denies.

Meds: Suspected Warfarin. Aspirin. Ibuprofen, occasional.

FamH: Mother—deceased, smoking-related; father—deceased, heart disease; brother—diabetes.

Physical Examination: Indicate only pertinent positive and negative findings related to the patient's chief complaint.

VS Stable. Elevated blood pressure noted.

Lymph nodes: Moderate generalized lymphadenopathy.

Lung: Clear to auscultation. No rhonchi, rales, or wheezes.

Heart: Regular, rate, and rhythm.

Abdomen: Soft, nontender. +bowel sounds. No hepatomegally. +splenomegally. Neg Murphy's sign. Neg rebound ttp.

Skin: Large macular ecchymosis on arms and on anterior shins. Right hip ecchymotic lesion approximately 5x6 cm. All lesions non blanchable. No ttp. Minimal skin breaks on hands.

Differential Diagnosis: In order of likelihood (with 1 being the most likely), list up to 5 potential or possible diagnoses for this patient's presentation (in many cases, fewer than 5 diagnoses are likely)	Diagnostic Work-up: List immediate plans (up to 5) for further diagnostic work-up
1. Leukemia (CLL, CML, AML)	1. CBC with differential
2. Warfarin medication effect	2. Coagulation panel (PT, aPTT, INR)
3. Multiple myeloma	3. Basic metabolic panel including electrolytes, renal function, and glucose.
4. Lymphoma	4. Liver enzyme panel with LDH
5. Thrombotic thrombocytopenic purpura (TTP)	5. Stool occult blood testing

1. Opening Scenario

Carrie Westermark, a 22-year-old pregnant female, comes to the office with burning when she urinates for the last 4 days.

2. Vital Signs

BP: 120/78 mmHg

Temp: 101.1° F (38.4° C)

HR: 78/minute, regular

RR: 16/minute

3. Examinee Tasks

1. Obtain a focused history.

2. Perform a relevant physical examination. (Do not perform breast, pelvic/genital, or rectal examination.)

3. Discuss your initial diagnostic impression and your work-up plan.

4. After leaving the room, complete your patient note on the given form.

Are the Vital Signs Stable?

Subjective

Knock; enter. Introduce yourself, and place the first signpost.

"Hello Ms. Westermark, nice to meet you, I'm Dr. Banebridge. I understand you've been having some trouble urinating lately. Please tell me about that."

"Hi doctor, nice to meet you. I've been having some **burning when I pee**. I'm also **pregnant**, as you can see—25 weeks now. My doctor told me to come in if this happens."

"Ok. How long has this been going on?"

"About **4 days** or so. It hurts when I start to pee, but it's better by the end. I mean, I know it sounds weird to talk about, but.... Is that anything to worry about?"

"Well, considering your pregnancy, yes, that's a symptom we do want to know about. It could indicate an infection, which is important to determine when you're pregnant. Do you have any other symptoms such as feeling hot?"

"Yeah, I felt like I've had a **fever since yesterday**. I don't know if it's the pregnancy hormones or something, but I've felt really hot. I **sweat through my sheets** last night in bed which I've never done before. But then again, you know, I had these really extreme mood shifts at the beginning of my pregnancy, so I think some of that is my weird hormones."

"It looks like you have a fever by your vital signs that the nurse just took, as well. That's unusual and, again, something we are interested in knowing about when you're pregnant. How about other problems, such as having to go to the bathroom a lot lately?"

"**Yeah**, that's almost a constant. I'm always in the bathroom. My doctor said I should expect a little of that because the baby's getting bigger. **I just figured that was it**."

"That can have a lot to do with it. How often would you say you go to the bathroom to urinate?"

"Oh, about **10 or 15 times a day**. It's really increased since the baby's gotten bigger. Since it burns to go, it's kind of miserable."

"I can imagine. How about a feeling of urgency when you have to go? That is, when you feel like you have to go, do you have to go immediately, or do you have a feeling of not being able to make it in time?"

"**Yeah**, that's been there since it started burning."

"Ok. And how about any blood in your urine? Have you noticed that?"

"**No**, it's been kind of dark lately, but I wouldn't say blood."

"Alright. Have you had any other symptoms, like back pain?"

"**Yeah**, my **back's** been hurting, too. It hurts when I bend over or do anything. I've had back problems before, though. My doctor said I had a spasm once when I saw her about 6 months ago for it. Now I'm pregnant, and I figured it was because of the baby, too. I got a pamphlet that said it could happen."

"That's true. Some back pain is expected as the baby gets bigger. I'll examine you in a few minutes and try to determine if that's it. Have you had other symptoms like nausea or vomiting?"

"**No**, I haven't had that since my first trimester. That was bad, though."

"Some people can get some of that sick feeling early on. I can only imagine how that feels. Did you take any medication because of that feeling?"

"**Yeah**, my doctor gave me some **promethizine**. I haven't taken that in quite a few months, though."

"How about a decrease in appetite lately?"

"**Yeah**, I **haven't eaten as much** the last few days. I'm much less hungry lately. My mother-in-law keeps telling me to eat more but…I don't know…I just don't feel like eating lately."

"Ok. Let me ask a few questions about your pregnancy, if you don't mind. How many times have you been pregnant?"

"Oh, this is the **first time**. My husband and I had been trying for 4 months to get pregnant."

"When is your due date?"

"It's April 9th."

When a patient reports frequency, it's important to know how many times per day. Relative frequency, especially when pregnant, may not be a symptom of anything worrisome.

Careful physical exam can delineate the critical difference between back pain and CVA tenderness.

When a pregnant patient is being evaluated, always check basic pregnancy data, such as date of last menstrual period (LMP) and due date.

"And when was your last menstrual period?"

"It started on the 4th of July this year."

"Great. And you mentioned you had some nausea and vomiting early on, which might be expected. Have there been any other problems with this pregnancy?"

"**Nope**, it's been great. My family says I'm glowing. I've really not had any problems."

"Have you felt the baby kick yet?"

"**Yeah**, I've felt it for about 2 weeks. It's really great."

"That's wonderful. How about the last few days?"

"Oh, **yeah**, I feel him or her kicking all the time. We don't know the sex yet."

"Ok. Have you had anything you might think is a contraction?"

"Oh, no."

"Any episodes of vaginal bleeding or unusual discharge?"

"**No**, I have a little **more discharge** than usual, though. My doctor said that's expected. I try to keep clean."

"Is the discharge the normal mucous, or is it another color?"

"**Yeah**, that's the thing, it's kind of **off-color** a little. Maybe a little darker. Not yellow but darker. And honestly, it **smells kind of bad**."

"Is it a white, almost cottage cheese-type consistency?"

"**No**, not really. Just **off-color**."

"Ok. I'd like to ask some personal questions about your sexual activity, if you don't mind. Are you sexually active now?"

"Sure, I don't mind. **Yeah**."

"Do you have a monogamous relationship? That is, do you each have only each other for partners?"

"Oh **yeah**, we're monogamous and married."

"When was the last time you had sex?"

"About a **week ago**, I guess."

"Do you have any problems with sex, such as pain?"

"Well, **kind of**. It sometimes **hurts in the beginning** a little."

"How long has it hurt?"

"Well, maybe a couple of **weeks** now. Maybe it's nothing."

"Have you had any sexually transmitted diseases in your life?"

"**No**."

"Do you know if your husband has?"

"He **hasn't** either."

"Ok. Have you ever had a yeast infection?"

"**No**, I don't think so."

"Alright. Let me ask about other symptoms. Have you had a recent illness?"

During the interview with a pregnant patient, always ask four key questions:
Vaginal bleeding?
Vaginal discharge?
Fetal movements felt?
Contractions felt?

Sexual history is important in a pregnant female suspected of infection. Go as in-depth as needed.

"I had a **cold about 2 weeks ago**. It was kind of miserable because I didn't want to take anything because of the baby."

"Ok. Do you still have any symptoms from that?"

"Well, I still have a **cough**. When I saw my doctor at my last pregnancy visit she said the cough can hold on for a while."

"That's true. Do you cough up anything when you cough?"

"**No**. In the beginning I did, but it's just an irritating **dry cough** now."

"You'd said earlier that you'd felt like you had a fever. Does that mean you've felt hot with body aches?"

"**Yeah**, when I have a fever I feel like I have a lot of **body aches**. Like I don't want to get out of bed. And I feel hot. That's what I've felt like lately. And I, kind of, sweat a lot at night. It was a whole lot last night."

"That's especially hard isn't it? How about chest congestion?"

"**Not** anymore."

"Have you had any other symptoms, such as headache or vision changes?"

"**No.**"

"Any unusual thirst lately?"

"**Nothing** more than normal."

"How about any weight loss recently? You should be gaining weight, but have you lost any?"

"**No**, I've been gaining steadily. I check every day. I've gained 15 lbs since the beginning. I'm kind of worried about being able to lose it once I deliver."

"Well, some people have some problem with that, but it can be easier than you think. Alright, how about any other health problems in your life? Have you seen the doctor for anything else?"

"When I was **16 years old,** I got onto **birth control** to control my periods. And when I was **9 years old,** I **broke my leg** when I was skiing. Nothing else though."

"Ok. How about any surgeries?"

"**Nope.**"

"Do you smoke, or are you around anyone that smokes?"

"**No**, nobody."

"Do you drink alcohol, or have you during this pregnancy?"

"**No**, not at all. My husband and I had been trying for a while, so I quit drinking a long time ago. I didn't want to hurt the baby."

"Good choice. Are you allergic to anything?"

"**No**, nothing."

"What medications are you on?"

"I'm taking the **prenatal vitamins**. I take an occasional **Tylenol** for small aches or pains but nothing else. I took two Tylenol last night, actually. I helped a little maybe."

"Alright. When was the last Tylenol dose you took?"

"Oh, maybe, about 3:00 this morning. I thought it would help with the hot feeling. I don't know."

Signpost for the Physical Exam

"Ok. I'd like to do a physical exam now, if you don't mind. Just let me wash my hands. It looks like your **vital signs are normal,** so please let me first listen to your heart and lungs…"

Objective

Points for Every Exam:

- Wash hands.
- Comment on vital signs, even if normal.
- Tell the patient where you are going to examine and disrobe.
- Do not repeat painful maneuvers.

Physical Exam:

Perform a focused physical, by system, from the head down.

System	Exam elements	Findings in this patient
Lungs	Auscultate the posterior lung fields. Make sure to listen to 6 points on the back.	No wheezes or rales. Mild scattered rhonchi in the left lung base.
Abdomen	Observe the abdomen for discoloration or unusual masses. Palpate the abdomen, asking if she is having pain in each quadrant. Check for tenderness over the bladder. Measure the uterus from the pubic symphysis to the superior edge of the fundus. Comment on findings, such as tenderness affecting other areas of the abdomen or abdominal guarding.	Normal appearance, normal bowel sounds. Mild tenderness over the bladder region. No masses. Fundal height approximately 25 cm. No palpable contractions. No guarding or uterine tenderness.
Back	Observe for spasm and palpate the midspine and perispinal musculature for tenderness. Check for costovertebral angle tenderness by percussion.	Moderate right CVA tenderness by gentle percussion. No spasm noted.
Genital/pelvic	Deferred	Deferred
Fetus	Assess fetal heart tones with a portable Doppler ultrasound device. Start just cephalad of the pubis and scan for fast tones distinct from the slow tones of the mother's own heartbeat.	Fetal heart tones found with heart rate of 160s bpm.

Continue to gather information as you do the physical exam. Ask about pertinent aspects of each system as you perform the exams. Comment aloud on any real or simulated abnormalities.

Example: *"Where do you normally get your menstrual cramping when it comes on?"*

Example: *"When you sometimes get constipated, does it hurt in this area?"*

End of Case

End by explaining you have several ideas of what could be wrong and could cause these symptoms. Tell the patient the first two diagnoses on your differential list and the major tests you'd now like to perform.

Example: *"Ms. Westermark, there are a few things that are concerning about what's going on with you today. First, because you're pregnant, I would like to treat you more conservatively than other people. But second, it's fairly likely that you may have a kidney infection. That's when an infection travels up from you lower urinary tract to your kidneys. This is an especially concerning situation in a pregnant person, because I want to make sure it doesn't get more serious. This could, however, also be from an infection of your vagina or cervix. For that possibility, I'd like to do a pelvic exam and take some tests today. The exam is much like a pap smear, but the* *samples will be analyzed for signs of bacteria rather than cancer. Otherwise, the exam is very similar. As well as these tests, I'd like to get some blood and urine from you to determine if an infection may be present. Please allow me to step out now and arrange these tests with my nurse.*

Before I go, is there any other aspect of your health care we haven't already discussed? Ok then, thank you."

PATIENT NOTE

History: Include significant positives and negatives from history of present illness, past medical history, review of system(s), social history, and family history.

HPI: 22 y/o G1P0 female at 25 0/7 wks pregnancy c/o fever and burning when she urinates. Symptoms include dysuria, frequency, and urgency beginning approximately 4 days ago. Fever and body aches started in the last 24 hours accompanied by night sweats last night. The patient endorses current and historic back pain. Patient endorses fetal movement, denies contractions or vaginal bleeding. She does report "off-color" vaginal discharge and mild dysparunia.

ROS: +dry cough, denies vision changes, denies overt thirst. O/w noncontributory.

Meds: Prenatal vitamins. Occasional Tylenol.

PMH: Recent cold like symptoms ending 2 wks ago. Fracture leg.

PSH: None.

Smoking: Denies.

Alcohol use: Denies.

Allergies: NKA.

Physical Examination: Indicate only pertinent positive and negative findings related to the patient's chief complaint.

VS stable, normal. Increased temperature noted.

Lungs: Clear to auscultation except for mild rhonchi at left lung base. No wheezes,, or rales.

Abdomen: Soft, nontender. Normal bowel sounds. Fundal height 25 cm. Mild tenderness over bladder. No guarding or uterine tenderness.

Back: Positive CVA tenderness on right side.

Differential Diagnosis: In order of likelihood (with 1 being the most likely), list up to 5 potential or possible diagnoses for this patient's presentation (in many cases, fewer than 5 diagnoses are likely)	Diagnostic Work-up: List immediate plans (up to 5) for further diagnostic work-up
1. Pyelonephritis	1. Pelvic exam with gonorrhea/Chlamydia DNA probes, KOH and wet prep mounts
2. Urinary tract infection	2. CBC with differential
3. Vaginal infection: bacterial vaginosis or trichomonas	3. Urine analysis and culture
4. Vaginal yeast infection	
5. Pneumonia	

1. Opening Scenario

Jose Montego, a 45-year-old male, presents to the clinic for evaluation of blood in his urine for the last month.

2. Vital Signs

BP: 128/86 mmHg

Temp: 98.8° F (37.1° C)

HR: 66/minute, regular

RR: 12/minute

3. Examinee Tasks

1. Obtain a focused history.

2. Perform a relevant physical examination. (Do not perform breast, pelvic/genital, or rectal examination.)

3. Discuss your initial diagnostic impression and your work-up plan.

4. After leaving the room, complete your patient note on the given form.

Are the Vital Signs Stable?

Subjective

Knock; enter. Introduce yourself, and place the first signpost.

"Hello Mr. Montego, I'm Dr. Mills. I understand you've been having some blood in your urine. Please tell me more about that."

"Hey doc. Yeah, I've been **bleeding on my underwear** for about a **month**. It's only happened a **few times,** but I wake up or whatever and see these blood stains on my underwear. Its kind of weird, you know? It's freaking me out."

"That must be strange. How long have you been seeing this blood?"

"It's been about a **month**. It doesn't happen every day, but it happens, maybe, a **couple times a week**. And when it happens, I'll go to the bathroom and my urine is, like, **dark or sort of orange**, you know?"

When clarification is needed, using analogies to common items is often useful. Always try to put your clarification in a vernacular the patient may understand.

"Are there any clots in your underwear or urine?"

"What do you mean clots?"

"I'm sorry. I mean small specs or clumps of solid blood. Blood that is a sort of a jello consistency rather than liquid. Larger ones or you may see only small specs in your urine."

"Oh, **no**. It's not like that. It's just a spot or two on my underwear. I wear white briefs so I can tell pretty well."

"Has this gotten worse over the month, or is it about the same?"

"It's gotten **worse**. I came in because it happened **every day now for about 10 days**. Just a little, but it's there. Like I said, **it's freaking me out**."

"I can imagine it's an odd thing to have to deal with. I'd like to ask you some more questions about it, then we'll do some testing. I think this will give me the best way to figure out what's going on and then we can find the best way to treat it. Ok?"

"Yeah, that's what I'm here for."

"Alright. Do you have any pain when you urinate?"

"**No**, it doesn't hurt. And it's almost always **only in the morning** that I see the real orange pee. When I drink more, it goes away a little."

"How about any pain in your abdomen?"

"Nope, nothing lately."

"Have you had any other unusual penile discharge?"

"Uh, **no**. Nothing else."

"Are you sexually active?"

"**Yeah.**"

"Ok. With men, women, or both?"

"**Women** only, doc. I have a girlfriend."

When taking a sexual history, a statement of acknowledgment of the personal nature of the questions often helps the patient relax.

"I can understand these questions may be a little personal. They're necessary for me to fully understand if you're at risk for a sexually transmitted disease. Are you monogamous with your partner?"

"Yeah, she's the only one I've been with for **7 years now**. We live together and have a son."

"Ok. Have you had any other pain in your genital region, such as your testicles or bladder?"

"**No**, not at all. I had a **vasectomy** 4 years ago now. That was right after our son was born. That was the last time I really had any pain down there. This blood doesn't hurt at all."

"Did you have any complications with that vasectomy?"

"**No**, it went fine. Some time on the couch, then it was ok."

"Have you had any blood in your semen?"

"I **don't know**, I never check. I don't think so."

"Have you ever had a sexually transmitted disease?"

"**No**, never."

"How many sexual partners have you had in your life?"

"I've had **six**, including my girlfriend. I married three of them. Sometimes it just doesn't work out. Women are nuts sometimes. You must know what I mean?"

"Well, it's very easy to have problems in any relationship. Have you ever had any other problems, such as kidney stones or prostate problems?"

"**No**. Never had stones or prostate stuff."

"When you urinate, do you ever have a problem starting a stream?"

"Well, like sometimes when I try to go, it's **hard to get it going**. I can after I stand there for a while, but it's kind of annoying because I have to wait."

"Yeah. Do you ever finish urinating and feel like there's still some that's left in your bladder?"

"**No**, not really. That's ok."

"How about the feeling that when you have to go to the bathroom to urinate, you really, really have to go quickly?"

"**Nope**."

"Do you ever urinate when you don't mean to?"

"**No**, not really."

"Do you ever get up at night to urinate?"

"Oh, **yeah**. That's been all my life. I get up **once or maybe twice**. That **hasn't changed**."

"Do you have anything else in your past medical history that you've seen the doctor for? Especially anything you've spent the night in the hospital for?"

"**No**, I don't like doctors. No offense. I don't go unless I have to. I've never been in the hospital, except when I was a kid. I had my **tonsils out**."

"Speaking of surgeries, is the tonsillectomy the only one you've had?"

"That's it, thank goodness."

"Have you ever had kidney stones?"

"**No**, never."

"Has your family ever had any major medical problems?"

"My dad has **Alzheimer's** disease. He's living with my sister. My mom lives alone because they got a divorce. She has some sort of **thyroid** gland problem. She takes **pills** for it every day. Otherwise, my sister and I are both good."

"Has anyone in your family had kidney stones?"

"**No**, nobody."

"How about any type of cancer?"

"**I don't think so**. I would know about that."

"Ok. Do now or have you ever used tobacco?"

"**No**, I never did. I have a lot of friends that do, but I never liked it."

Patients may make derogatory statements then seek common ground with the physician. This is meant to find familiarity and commonality; however, it's important you keep your professional distance from these statements. But also be careful not to alienate the patient for making them.

If possible, try to smoothly transition from one related question to another. This makes the patient more at ease with the interview.

"How about drinking alcohol?"

"I did about 15 years ago. I'm a **recovering alcoholic**. I **never touch it anymore**. That's part of the treatment. I never touch it. Sober for 15 years now."

"Congratulations on being sober that long. That's quite an accomplishment."

"Thanks. I don't even want to anymore."

"How about any other drugs? Now or in the past?"

"**Nope**, the bottle was my drug."

"Do you take any medications now?"

"No, I don't see the doctor long enough. I don't like pills either."

"How about over-the-counter medications, such as Motrin or Naprosyn?"

"I take a **Tylenol** or **Motrin** from time to time. I'd say, maybe once a week. Not much though."

"What do you take it for?"

"A **headache** here or there. Or some **aches or pains**. I'm a roofer so it's hard work sometimes."

"I can imagine that's very physically demanding. Do these headaches go away with these medications?"

"Oh yeah. They're nothing big, just every now and then."

"Ok. Do you ever get lightheaded or have any problems with balance?"

"**No**, no."

"How about any pain in your chest or trouble breathing?"

"**No**. None of those."

"Do you ever have trouble with digestion? Like diarrhea or throwing up?"

"**No**, unless I get the flu."

"You mentioned aches and pains. Is that work-related, or do you get those pains when you're not at work, too?"

"Oh, it's all **related to work**. You know, if I have a rough day or something. Nothing big."

Signpost for the Physical Exam

"Ok. I'd like to do a physical exam now, if you don't mind. Just let me **wash my hands**. First I'd like to examine your lungs, then I'll step out so you may change into a gown. I'd also like to do a genital and prostate exam…"

Objective

Points for Every Exam:

- Wash hands.
- Comment on vital signs, even if normal.
- Tell the patient where you are going to examine and disrobe.
- Do not repeat painful maneuvers.

Physical Exam:

Perform a focused physical, by system, from the head down.

System	Exam elements	Findings in this patient
Lungs	Auscultate the posterior and side lung fields. Make sure to listen to 6 points on the posterior lung fields and 1 on each lateral lung field.	Clear to auscultation. No wheezes, rhonchi, or rales
Abdomen	Purcuss the costovertebral angles (CVA) for pain. Listen for BSs. Gently palpate all 4 quadrants and epigastrim. Listen for abdominal bruit's.	Normal BSs. No ttp, including over epigastrim. No masses. No abdominal bruit's. No CVA tenderness.

Continue to gather information as you do the physical exam. Comment aloud on any real or simulated abnormalities.

Example: *"Have you had a cough lately?"*

Example: *"Does it hurt when I press here* [while applying direct pressure of the bladder region]*?"*

End of Case

End by explaining you have several ideas of what could be wrong and could cause these symptoms. Tell the patient the first two diagnoses on your differential list and the major tests you'd now like to perform.

Example: *"Mr. Montego, the blood in your urine may be to the result of several different causes. The first task of finding out what might be wrong is to figure out where the blood is coming from. In men above the age of 40, the blood may possibly be from the bladder and may be caused by a cancer there. That's one possibility and the most concerning, although this would still be a rare cause of your bleeding. It may also be coming from your prostate, or the gland that produces much of the liquid part of semen. Your symptom of having to strain to start a stream of urine is not uncommon for a condition many men have called benign prostatic hyperplasia. This is a noncancerous enlargement of the prostate gland that sometimes can cause bleeding into the urine. Yet other sources of bleeding could include the kidneys themselves or result from almost anywhere along the urinary system because of tiny kidney stones or infection. These are broad categories of illnesses, and I want you to know I can't tell yet which is the most likely. To find out, I'd like to order several tests that will require some urine, blood, and for you to undergo another procedure to examine the bladder and the tube it exits through your penis. This is called 'cystoscopy' and involves using a very small camera to actually look at these areas. I'd also like to do a genital and prostate exam on you today to evaluate for some of these possibilities. Please allow me to step out and arrange these tests and give you a chance to change into your gown.*

Is there any other aspect of your health care we haven't already discussed? Ok then, thank you."

PATIENT NOTE

History: Include significant positives and negatives from history of present illness, past medical history, review of system(s), social history, and family history.

HPI: 45 y/o male with c/o hematuria and bloody penile discharge x 1 month. Gross hematuria noted with gradual onset happening 2–3 times/week, which progressed to every day x prior 10 days. Blood noted on underclothes without clots. He denies prior STDs, dysuria, nonbloody penile discharge, pain in his testicles or urinary tract. Positive straining when starting urination although denies frequency, urgency, post void residual, or nocturia. Denies fever, pulmonary symptoms, abdominal symptoms, or prior episodes.

PMH: Occasional headache, muscular aches.

PSH: Vasectomy—s/p x 4 years.

Tobacco: Denies.

EtOH: Recovering alcoholic. Sober X 15 years.

Drugs: Denies.

SexHx: Monogamous X 7 years. Denies prior STDs. Six sex partners in lifetime.

Meds: Occasional ibuprofen/Tylenol.

FamH: Mother—thyroid condition; father—Alzheimer's. No urolithiasis.

Physical Examination: Indicate only pertinent positive and negative findings related to the patient's chief complaint.

VS Stable.

Lungs: Clear to auscultation bilaterally. No wheezes, rubs, or rhonchi.

Abdomen: Normal bowel sounds. No ttp over all 4 quadrants and epigastrum. No masses. No abdominal bruit's. No CVA tenderness.

Differential Diagnosis: In order of likelihood (with 1 being the most likely), list up to 5 potential or possible diagnoses for this patient's presentation (in many cases, fewer than 5 diagnoses are likely)	Diagnostic Work-up: List immediate plans (up to 5) for further diagnostic work-up
1. Prostatic bleeding	1. Genital and digital rectal (prostate) exam
2. Urinary tract infection	2. Urine analysis and culture
3. Urolithiasis	3. CT scan abdomen/pelvis
4. Glomerulonephritis	4. Cystoscopy
5. Bladder malignancy	5. Basic metabolic panel (BUN, creatinine, sodium, potassium, chloride, bicarbonate, glucose)

30. Testicular Mass

1. Opening Scenario

Michael Johansson, a 30-year-old male, presents to the physician's clinic with complaints of right testicular mass.

2. Vital Signs

BP: 126/62 mmHg

Temp: 99.0° F (37.2° C)

HR: 66/minute, regular

RR: 16/minute

3. Examinee Tasks

1. Obtain a focused history.

2. Perform a relevant physical examination. (Do not perform breast, pelvic/genital, or rectal examination.)

3. Discuss your initial diagnostic impression and your work-up plan.

4. After leaving the room, complete your patient note on the given form.

Are the Vital Signs Stable?

Subjective

Knock; enter. Introduce yourself, and place the first signpost.

"Hi, Mr. Johansson, I'm Dr. Drexlor. I understand you've recently found a mass on your testicle. Please tell me more about it."

"Hi, doctor. Yeah, I've found a **mass** on the **right** one. I don't know how long it's been there, but I **noticed it in the shower about 3 days ago**. It **doesn't hurt**; it just makes me nervous because I don't think I've ever felt it before."

"I can understand how it might make you feel uneasy. It's best to come in and have this sort of finding checked out. Where exactly is the lump?"

Transition Statement of empathy

"I found it sort of on the top. It's hard to explain but sort of right near the top. I don't know. I mean, I don't want to come in for every little thing, you know? I just figure, if something's there that wasn't there before, I'm going to get it looked at. Anyway, it's probably nothing."

"I completely agree with you. It's much safer to come in and get checked out than wonder if you didn't. Is it right on the testicle or within the scrotum itself?"

"I **think** it's on the **testicle**. It's hard to really say but if it's not on the testicle, its **right near** it."

"You said that it isn't painful; has it ever been?"

"**No**, it feels a little funny because I've been focusing so much on it, but it's never been painful, really."

"Has it ever swollen or has the area ever had redness to it?"

"**Not really**."

"How big is the lump itself, when you compare it to the testicle?"

"It's probably the size of a **bee**. Maybe a **pea** at the largest. You know?"

"Ok. That's good. What would you say it feels like? That is, is it hard or soft?"

"It's pretty **soft**. I mean, I can squeeze it sort of… it's not really hard. Doesn't hurt."

"Ok. Have you ever had surgery on your genitals?"

> Prior genital surgery should be fully explored in a patient with a genital-related complaint.

"Yeah, I had a **vasectomy 2 years ago**. It went fine. I thought that'd be the last time for anything like that. I don't like doctors down there, you know?"

"I can understand that. Did you have any complications from that surgery?"

"**No**, I stayed off my feet for a few days, and it was sore, but there weren't any problems."

"Ok. Did you have a follow-up sperm sample after the operation?"

"**Yeah**, it was negative. It showed I'm shooting blanks."

"Have you had any trauma to the area in your life?"

"Well, **no**. I've been **hit there every now and again** by a football or whatever, but nothing I wouldn't expect is normal."

"Alright. How about any burning when you urinate?"

"**No**, nothing like that."

"Have you ever had a sexually transmitted disease?"

"**No**, never. I've been married now for 14 years. There's never been that kind of problem in our marriage."

"Ok. Just so I can collect the right information, has your wife ever had a sexually transmitted disease?"

"**Nope**."

"Ok. Have you had any unusual discharge from your penis?"

"**No**, it's normal."

"Have you had any noticable blood in your urine or semen?"

"**Nope**."

"I understand you found this lump a few days ago, but have you had a recent fever?"

"Nah."

"How about feeling tired or having body aches?"

"Well…not really. I feel alright lately."

"Anything like nausea or diarrhea or feeling overly hot or cold?"

"Honestly, I've felt fine."

"Alright, let me ask a few questions about your past medical history. What have you seen the doctor for in your life?"

"Well, there was that **vasectomy** a few years ago. I also **broke my thumb** when I was 27 years old. It didn't heal right, so I had to have it **operated** on. Other than that, I got my cholesterol checked a few months ago, and everything's fine."

"When you were born, did your mother ever tell you that you had what's called an 'undescended testicle' or a testicle that didn't come all the way down into your scrotum?"

"**No**, no one ever said anything like that to me. I mean, I'd remember that."

"Ok. Are those operations for the vasectomy and your thumb the only surgeries you've ever had?"

"**Yeah**, that's it."

"How about any medications—are you on any?"

"**No**, I don't even take Tylenol if I don't have to. I hate taking pills."

"Do you smoke or use tobacco?"

"I **dip** about **half a can** a day. I don't smoke, though."

"How about drink alcohol?"

"I have a **glass of wine** with dinner on the **weekends**. I've got three kids at home, and I don't drink much anymore. I've settled down."

"That sounds reasonable. Has anyone in your family had any major disease?"

"Well, my **mom** had a **hysterectomy** for **fibroids,** and then she had a part of her colon taken out for **diverticulitis**. That was a while ago. My **dad** died 3 years ago now in a car **accident**. My brother's in Florida and has **high blood pressure,** but that's it. Otherwise, nothing."

> History of cryptorchidism increases the chances of malignancy >20-fold. Although unusual, it's worth specifically asking about.

Signpost for the Physical Exam

"Ok. I'd like to do a physical exam now, if you don't mind. I'll step out while I ask you to change into a gown for a genital exam. Before I go, I'd like to examine your lymph nodes in your groin, if you don't mind. Just let me **wash my hands**…"

Objective

Points for Every Exam:

- Wash hands.
- Comment on vital signs, even if normal.
- Tell the patient where you are going to examine and disrobe.
- Do not repeat painful maneuvers.

Physical Exam:

Perform a focused physical, by system, from the head down.

System	Exam elements	Findings in this patient
Inguinal area	Check for enlarged inguinal lymph nodes or palpable masses. Don't perform a genital or inguinal hernia exam.	Normal, no lymphadenopathy
Genital	Deferred	Deferred

Continue to gather information as you do the physical exam. Comment aloud on any real or simulated abnormalities.

Example: "*Do you have pain when I press here* [pressing on the inguinal area]*?*"

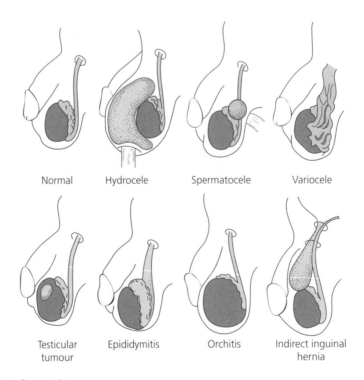

FIGURE 30.1 Diagnosis of scrotal masses.

Reprinted with permission from Longmore & Wilkinson. *Oxford Handbook of Clinical Medicine*, 6th ed. Oxford University Press, 2004.

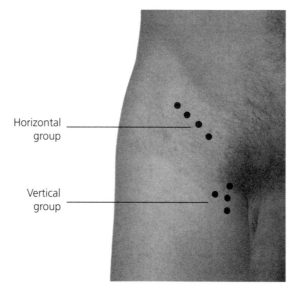

FIGURE 30.2 Diagrammatic representation of the inguinal lymph nodes.

Reprinted with permission from Thomas & Monahan. *Oxford Handbook of Clinical Examination and Practical Skills.* Oxford University Press, 2007.

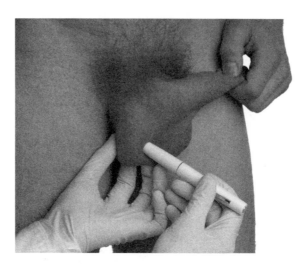

FIGURE 30.3 Attempt to transilluminate any swelling by shining a small flashlight through it. The room should be darkened.

Reprinted with permission from Thomas & Monahan. *Oxford Handbook of Clinical Examination and Practical Skills.* Oxford University Press, 2007.

End of case

End by explaining you have several ideas of what could be wrong and could cause these symptoms. Tell the patient the first two diagnoses on your differential list and the major tests you'd now like to perform.

Example: *"Mr. Johansson, before doing a physical exam and feeling the lump in your testicle myself, there are a few possibilities that come to mind. First, I think its best go evaluate cancer of the testicle, which can sometimes be felt as a lump. Simply feeling the lump is the first step, but I'll also want to obtain an ultrasound of the* testicle to actually look at it. An ultrasound should be fairly pain-free and involves simply placing a probe onto the surface of the scrotum and looking at the testicle on a screen. That's the best way to tell if you might need a biopsy or other action. As well as the ultrasound, I'd like to be able to get some blood work to evaluate some factors that may be given off by this type of cancer, if it actually is cancer. Remember, cancer is a rare possibility, but because it's the most serious, I'd like to be safe and get you evaluated for it. Another possibility is that this could be a benign lump called a "sperm granuloma" that commonly forms after a vasectomy. This is basically a small piece of scar tissue formed by a small inflammatory reaction from sperm leakage out of the end of the tube that normally carries sperm to the penis. Because this tube was cut during your vasectomy, sometimes the sperm causes a slight inflammatory reaction, and you may feel this as a lump.

Is there any other aspect of your health care we haven't already discussed? Ok then, thank you."

PATENT NOTE

History: Include significant positives and negatives from history of present illness, past medical history, review of system(s), social history, and family history.

HPI: 30 y/o male with newly discovered right testicular mass x 3 days. Mass is reportedly located at superior pole of the right testicle and is soft in nature. No tenderness or pain. No history overt trauma. Vasectomy 2 years ago reported as uncomplicated. Denies urinary symptoms such as dysuria, penile d/c. Currently in monogamous marriage x 14 years. No prior STDs.

PMH: Fractured thumb.

PSH: Vasectomy—2 years ago.

Tobacco: Dips ½ can per day. No smoking.

Alcohol use: Occasional.

Meds: Denies.

FamH: Mother—fibroids, diverticulitis; father—deceased, trauma; brother—hypertension.

Physical Examination: Indicate only pertinent positive and negative findings related to the patient's chief complaint.

VS Stable.

Inguinal lymph nodes: No lymphadenopathy, mass, or tenderness.

Differential Diagnosis: In order of likelihood (with 1 being the most likely), list up to 5 potential or possible diagnoses for this patient's presentation (in many cases, fewer than 5 diagnoses are likely)	Diagnostic Work-up: List immediate plans (up to 5) for further diagnostic work-up
1. Sperm granuloma	1. Genital exam, including inguinal hernia exam
2. Testicular malignancy	2. Testicular ultrasound
3. Hydrocele	3. β-hCG
4. Varicocele	4. α-fetoprotein
5. Hernia	5.

1. Opening Scenario

Erin Rivera, a 28-year-old female, presents to the office with complaints of irregular periods for 2 months.

2. Vital Signs

BP:	138/72 mmHg
Temp:	98.9° F (37.2° C)
HR:	76/minute, regular
RR:	16/minute
Weight:	165 lb (75 kg)
Height:	5'2" (1.6 m)
BMI:	30.2 kg/m²

3. Examinee Tasks

1. Obtain a focused history.

2. Perform a relevant physical examination. (Do not perform breast, pelvic/genital, or rectal examination.)

3. Discuss your initial diagnostic impression and your work-up plan.

4. After leaving the room, complete your patient note on the given form.

Are the Vital Signs Stable?

Subjective

Knock; enter. Introduce yourself and place the first signpost.

"Hello Ms. Rivera, I'm Dr. Biggsby. I understand you've had irregular periods lately. Please tell me more about this?"

"Hi doctor. I've really been having some **weird periods**. I mean, I haven't had much of a period the last 2 months. When I'm not on my birth control pills, my periods are usually screwed up and I'm not regular, but it's been really messed up lately, and I am on it. I actually was put on **birth control** a **year ago** because they were so bad."

"Please tell me how they are irregular. When was the last time you had a period?"

"That was a **few weeks ago**. That is, I had bleeding then, but it was more like **spotting** here and there. It wasn't a real period. Then **last month** I just **spotted**, too. Last month it was a little more around the time I was supposed to have a period but not much more."

"When are you in your cycle now?"

"If I was going to have it, I **would be on my period now**. It should have **started yesterday**. I didn't though, not at all."

"How long is there usually between your periods?"

"Well, about **27 or 28 days**. Like I said, when I'm on my birth control."

"Have you had other symptoms of your period such as, perhaps, cramping?"

"Yeah, I got **cramps** a few weeks ago. It was only a few here and there, and it didn't stop me from going to work but it was there."

"Can you characterize the bleeding? That is, does the flow appear like bright red blood or is it darker like menstrual flow?"

"I guess it's **like a period**. I use **tampons** so I don't check much."

"How long did the bleeding last during the episode that was a couple weeks ago?"

"It was about **2 days**. I felt like it was going to be longer because of the cramps, but that was all."

"How about the time before that? Last month?"

"That time it lasted maybe **3 to 4 days**. Some **small cramping** with that one.

"And how long are your periods normally? That is, when they are regular and you're on birth control?"

"They're about **5 days**. **Maybe 4 days** but usually not shorter than that. The flow is kind of **constant**, too, you know? The last few months it's been a little, then a lot, then a little. Just more **irregular**."

"Ok. You stated you had irregular periods and are subsequently on birth control pills now; what pills are you taking?"

"They're called **Ortho-Novum**. I've always been on those. They work well, but sometimes they're hard to remember. But I've never had a problem with them with my migraines so I like them."

"Do they make your periods more regular?"

"Oh **yeah**. They're really good at that, but if I get off them, the periods are pretty irregular again."

"Have you recently skipped any pills?"

"I try to take them if I can as soon as I remember. I missed one when we went away for the weekend about a month ago. Last week I missed one too. If I miss one, I usually take it that night, though."

"Ok. I'd like to ask you some personal questions now about your sexual habits. Is that alright?"

Signpost the beginning of a potentially uncomfortable line of questioning such as the sexual history. This prepares the patient mentally for personal questions.

"Sure."

"Are you sexually active?"

"**Yeah**, I'm engaged, actually. Six months now, so yes."

"Oh, congratulations. That's always great to hear. Is it safe to assume you're monogamous, then?"

"**Yeah, we both are**."

"How many sexual partners have you had in your life?"

"**Three.**"

"Have you ever had a sexually transmitted disease?"

"**No**, I haven't."

"Do you know if your partners have ever had a sexually transmitted disease?"

"**I don't think so**. If they did, I would've probably broken up with them."

"Ok. Do you have any problems with sexual intercourse, like pain?"

"**No**, sex is ok. I don't have any problems."

"Other than the unusual bleeding, do you have any other vaginal discharge?"

"**No**, I know what a yeast infection feels like, and that's the only time I've had an unusual discharge."

"How long has it been since you had a yeast infection?"

"Well, it's been about **2 years**. I haven't had one in a long time."

"Do you often have bleeding after sex?"

"**No**, not at all."

"Do you have any other symptoms, like unusual nipple discharge?"

"**No,** I've never had anything come out of my nipples."

"Ok. I know you have migraine headaches. Have you had one lately?"

"**No**, I've been on the birth control, so it's been about **8 months** or so since I've had one."

"Any other problems like congestion in your chest or nausea or diarrhea lately?"

"**No**, no recent illnesses."

"Do you have any pain when you urinate?"

"**Nope**."

"How about feeling like you have to urinate more often than usual?"

"**No**, that's fine, too."

"Other than the Ortho-Novum, are you on any other medications?"

"I'm on **Celexa** for **depression**. I take one of those every day."

"Ok. Do you smoke now or have you in the past?"

"**No**, I used to smoke when I went out with my friends but stopped. I just don't like the way it makes my clothes smell."

"How about drinking?"

Pleasantries over simple things often deepen the patient–doctor relationship.

"Like I said, I go out with my friends every now and then, and we might have a **drink or two**. I don't do that much anymore, though, since I got engaged. I just don't like to party that much anymore."

"How many drinks per week do you have?"

"Any more? Maybe **one** if you average them all together. I really don't drink, though."

"Ok. Do you take any other drugs?"

"**No** not at all."

"How about any diet aids or supplements?"

"**No**, I just try to eat healthy."

"Alright. Let me ask about your past medical history. Have you seen the doctor for any major problems in your life? Especially anything for which you were required to spend the night in the hospital?"

"I saw my doctor for the **birth control** issue last year. I have my annual exam every year. I also have migraine headaches. Usually I can just take Motrin and try to sleep, but those are much less frequent since I've been on birth control."

"Do you take any other medicine for the headaches?"

"No, I tried **Imitrex** once, but it didn't do anything. I just take the **Motrin** and try to sleep, that's enough."

"Alright. Have you ever had an abnormal pap smear?"

"I did about **2 years ago**. We did pap smears more often and even did one of those scopes. Eventually, it **went away**, though."

"Ok. Have you ever been pregnant?"

Never, Never, get into a discussion over personal opinions on controversial subjects such as abortion, even if you may agree with the patient's views.

"When I was **15 years old** I got pregnant. I had an **abortion**, though. My parents and I agreed that it was the best thing to do. Other than that, no."

"Have you ever had any other type of procedure? Such as surgery?"

"**Nope**."

"Does anyone in your family have an inherited or major disease?"

"**Both my parents** have **diabetes**. They're both on medication for it. I'm an only child."

"Do your parents take insulin?"

Asking if relatives who have diabetes are on insulin may give a clue to which type. If they don't inject insulin or take pills, they most likely have type II. If they do inject insulin, more information is needed.

"**No**, they take the pills."

"Ok. Do your parents have any other health problems, such as heart disease or high blood pressure?"

"**No**, I don't think so."

Signpost for the Physical Exam

"Ok. I'd like to do a physical exam now, if you don't mind. Just let me **wash my hands.** I'd first like examine your thyroid gland…"

Objective

Points for Every Exam:

- Wash hands.
- Comment on vital signs, even if normal.
- Tell the patient where you are going to examine and disrobe.
- Do not repeat painful maneuvers.

Physical Exam:

Perform a focused physical, by system, from the head down.

System	Exam elements	Findings in this patient
Thyroid	Thyroid exam. Ask the patient to swallow while palpating the patient's anterior, inferior throat.	Normal

Continue to gather information as you do the physical exam. Comment aloud on any real or simulated abnormalities.

Example: *"Is there any pain when I feel your neck here?"*

End of Case

End by explaining you have several ideas of what could be wrong and could cause these symptoms. Tell the patient the first two diagnoses on your differential list and the major tests you'd now like to perform.

Example: *"Ms. Rivera, there are a number of things that may be causing your irregular periods. The first thing I'd like to find out is if you're pregnant because that can sometimes cause this type of bleeding. To find that out, there is a simple blood test we can do in the office today. Another reason for unusual bleeding may be an abnormality of the lower genital tract-like infection. For this, I'd like to do a pelvic exam today and obtain some swabs of your cervix for testing. These swabs can tell if sexually transmitted diseases or other infections such as yeast or parasites are present. Because you've had an abnormal pap in the past, I'd also like to get a pap smear at the same time. There are some other possibilities that I'd also like to test for by taking some blood samples. It'll be easiest if we do the pregnancy test and the other tests from the same blood so you don't have to be stuck in the arm more than once. I'd like to step out now and give you a chance to change into a gown. I'll also arrange these tests with my nurse.*

Is there any other aspect of your health care we haven't already discussed? Ok then, thank you."

PATIENT NOTE

History: Include significant positives and negatives from history of present illness, past medical history, review of system(s), social history, and family history.

HPI: 28 y/o female with complaints of irregular menses x 2 months. Pt states she is taking Ortho-Novum combination OCPs with otherwise normal menses on a 28-day cycle lasting a duration of approx 5 days. + occasional missed doses of OCP. + "spotting" bleeding x 4 days occurring 1 month ago. +vaginal bleeding 2 wks ago lasting 2 days and irregular. Both episodes accompanied by cramping c/w menses. Pt denies vaginal d/c, dysparunia, urinary symptoms, or prior STD. +Sex activity in reported monogamous male/female relationship.

PMH: Uncommon migraine type headaches. Depression. Prior yeast infection.

PSH: Intentional abortion age: 15 yrs.

POBHx: G1P0.

Tobacco: Denies.

EtOH: Occasional/social.

Drugs: Denies.

Meds: Ortho-Novum, Celexa, Motrin.

FamH: Both parents with likely type II diabetes controlled with oral medications. Otherwise noncontributory.

Physical Examination: Indicate only pertinent positive and negative findings related to the patient's chief complaint.

VS Stable.

Thyroid: Symmetric, nontender. No nodules or enlargement.

Differential Diagnosis: In order of likelihood (with 1 being the most likely), list up to 5 potential or possible diagnoses for this patient's presentation (in many cases, fewer than 5 diagnoses are likely)	Diagnostic Work-up: List immediate plans (up to 5) for further diagnostic work-up
1. Pregnancy	1. Pelvic and breast exams
2. Spontaneous abortion	2. β-HCG (qualitative)
3. Infection of the cervix or vagina	3. Gonorrhea/Chlamydia DNA probes and wet mount and KOH prep from cervical swabs.
4. Polycystic ovarian syndrome	4. TSH/free T4
5. Hyperprolactinemia	5. Prolactin level

1. Opening Scenario

Bobby Swennis, a 9-year-old male, presents to the physician's office with his mother for fever lasting 1 day.

2. Vital Signs

BP: 116/62 mmHg

Temp: 99.9° F (37.7° C)

HR: 78/minute, regular

RR: 16/minute

3. Examinee Tasks

1. Obtain a focused history.

2. Perform a relevant physical examination. (Do not perform breast, pelvic/genital, or rectal examination.)

3. Discuss your initial diagnostic impression and your work-up plan.

4. After leaving the room, complete your patient note on the given form.

This case involves a simulated child. The child patient is indicated upon entering the room.

Are the Vital Signs Stable?

Subjective

Knock; enter. Introduce yourself and place the first signpost.

"Hello Ms. Swennis, it's nice to see you today. This must be Bobby. How are you, Bobby? I'm Dr Nordman."

Bobby: "Fine."

"Ms. Swennis, I understand he's had an elevated temperature lately. Please tell me more about it."

> If a child is present, acknowledge them with a quick introduction or pleasantry. This puts both the parent and child at ease.

"Yes doctor, he had a fever **last night and all of yesterday**. He's been going out in the **cold weather** a lot lately after school, and I think he caught the **flu** or something."

"Ok. Have you taken his temperature at home?"

"Yeah, I took it and it said **102 degrees,** so I gave him some **Tylenol**. At least it helped him go to sleep."

"Where was that temperature taken?"

"I took it under his tongue."

"Ok. Has he complained of not feeling well other than this fever?"

"Well, he's said he has had a **sore throat,** but that's been for a while now. Like I said, he's gone outside a lot after school, and he's been having a **runny nose** for a little while, too. I think it's just not wearing his coat, but his last real **stuffy nose** was about 2 weeks ago when the **whole family** came down with the same thing. One of my other children brought it home from school, and you know how it is, it must've been passed it to the rest of us."

"I can imagine. That sort of thing gets passed from one person to the other quite easily. Has he said he has pain in his ears at all?"

"**No**, he hasn't had pain anywhere as far as I know. [Addressing the child] Do you hurt anywhere?"

Bobby: "**Huh, uh**."[indicating no]

"Bobby, can you tell me if your ears hurt?"

Bobby: "Huh, uh. Well, maybe a little. In 'dis one." [indicating his left ear]

"Ok. Does it hurt anywhere else? How about your throat?"

Bobby: "**No**."

"He tells me he has a **sore throat in the mornings,** but he hadn't acted like it all day. This past day he seemed to start feeling bad. I think it's the fever. He didn't want to go outside and play. He just looks run-down and **feels hot**."

"Did you take his temperature today?"

"Yeah, this morning it was **102.1 degrees**. I gave him some more **Tylenol** before we left for the appointment."

"Ok. Have there been any other problems such as nausea or vomiting?"

"No, he's been fine for that. He **didn't eat much dinner** last night but isn't throwing up."

"Has he had any diarrhea lately?"

"**No**, no diarrhea."

"You mentioned others in the house with a similar illness; who specifically?"

"I had it, my **husband** had it. His big **brother** and little **sister** also had it. Our baby is the only one that didn't get sick. Thank goodness."

"Well, thank goodness the baby didn't get sick. In Bobby, how about symptoms other than the sore throat, runny nose, picky eating, and fever? Anything else, like discharge from his ears?"

It's often relevant to ask where the temperature was taken as it can vary depending on the anatomic place of origin.

Children may respond in whatever way they perceive adults want them to answer.

"**No**, nothing else."

"Ok. Has he ever had an ear infection?"

"**Yes**, when he was a toddler he had about five in a row. The doctor said he would have put some ear tubes in but didn't because he stopped getting them."

"Wow, that is a lot. What about a bladder infection?"

"**No**, never that."

"Has he recently had any accidents or injuries?"

"**No**, he does pretty well besides a skinned knee from time to time. But that's been rare, really. Not recently."

"Has he ever seen the doctor for anything serious in his life? Especially anything for which he might have stayed the night in the hospital?"

"When he was about 2 years old he got an operation to put a **hernia** that was around his belly button back in. We took him home that night, though. **Nothing else**."

"Ok. Has he gotten all his vaccinations up to this point?"

"**Yeah**, he has."

"Ok. Let me ask a little about his home environment. Does anyone smoke in the home?"

"**No**, my husband quit with our first child. My parents smoke, but they only visit about twice per year. He's never around smoke."

"You had mentioned the two doses of Tylenol today and yesterday. Has he gotten any other doses of it?"

"**No**, that was the only thing I gave him. That worked so I didn't need anything else."

"Ok. How about anything else as far as medications?"

"**Nope**, he's not on anything else. I give him a chewable **multivitamin** with breakfast most days, but that's all."

"Has he ever had any type of developmental delay?"

"**No**, he's always been fine on his check-ups. His growth chart's been normal."

"Ok. How about allergies? Is he allergic to anything?"

"**Not** that we know of."

"Alright. Please tell me if there are any major diseases in the family. Is there anything that has occurred in your family that may affect him?"

"Um, **no**, not that I can think of. My parents and my husband's parents are both healthy. My mom thought she had cervical cancer last year, but it turned out to be nothing."

Signpost for the Physical Exam

"Ok. I'd like to do a physical exam now, if you don't mind. Just let me wash my hands. It looks like Bobby's **vital signs are normal,** although he has a

> When a child has an otherwise unexplained fever, try to isolate a possible source by system (i.e., URI, pneumonia, UTI, GI, etc.).

> Clarification of previously discussed points is important for complete history-taking. Completeness is more important than orderliness of the interview.

slightly increased temperature. I'd like to start out by looking in his throat with my penlight. Bobby, do you think I could take a look in your mouth for just a minute?..."

Objective

Points for Every Exam:

- Wash hands.
- Comment on vital signs, even if normal.
- Tell the patient where you are going to examine and disrobe.
- Do not repeat painful maneuvers.

Physical Exam:

Perform a focused physical, by system, from the head down.

System	Exam elements	Findings in this patient
HEENT	Eyes: Examine the external eyes, making sure to retract the lower lids. Observe constriction of the pupils. Ears: Use the otoscope with insufalator bulb to find the tympanic membrane and note erythema, retraction, bulging, immobility, altered light reflex, or discharge. Take your time with the insufalator bulb. Nose: Check each nostril with a simple otoscope cover. Throat: Use a tongue depressor and quickly observe the teeth, gums, anterior mouth and especially the posterior pharyngeal wall and tonsillar pillars.	Eyes: normal.PERRLA. Ears: left ear shows mild erythema and bulging. No discharge. Air/fluid level noted. Nose: normal without erythema. Throat: positive posterior pharyngeal erythema and moderate tonsillar swelling. Positive exudates.
Neck	Check for symmetry or lymphadenopathy of the cervical chains. Check Kernigs/Brudzinski's signs.	Shotty anterior cervical lymphadenopathy, negative Kernig's/Brudzinsky's. No nuchal rigidity.
Lungs	Auscultate the posterior lung fields. Make sure to listen to 6 points on the posterior fields. If rhonchi or rales are heard, test for egophony and tactile frematous.	Clear to auscultation bilaterally. No wheezes, rhonchi, or rales.
Skin	Ask the mother to help undress the patient, and observe the skin for rashes or focal areas of erythema. [simulated patient]. If only a live patient is provided, defer the exam.	Normal

Continue to gather information as you do the physical exam. Comment aloud on any real or simulated abnormalities.

Example: *[Addressing Bobby] "Does it hurt when you swallow?"*

Example: *"Gosh, when I look in your ears, I see some broccoli growing in there! Does that broccoli hurt!?"*

TABLE 32.1 Some Common Respiratory Conditions and Signs.

Condition	Age	Inspection	Auscultation
Bronchiolitis	<1 year	Pale, coryza, cough, recessions, tachypnoea	Wheeze and crackles throughout chest
Croup (laryngotracheobronchitis)	1–2 years	Stridor, hoarse voice, barking cough	Clear
Asthma	>1 year	Tachypnoea, recessions ± audible wheeze and use of accessory muscles	Wheeze, variable air entry throughout chest. Crackles in young children
Pneumonia	Infant	Tachypnoea, recessions, flushing due to fever, grunting	May be clear, reduced breath sounds over affected area, crackles
Pneumonia	Child	Tachypnoea, recessions, flushed, generally unwell	Abdominal pain (may be the only symptom), crackles and bronchial breathing over affected area

▶ ↑ respiratory rate and work of breathing are the most important signs of a lower respiratory tract infection in infancy, as sometimes palpation, percussion, and auscultation will be normal.

Reprinted with permission from Thomas & Monahan. *Oxford Handbook of Clinical Examination and Practical Skills.* Oxford University Press, 2007.

End of Case

End by explaining you have several ideas of what could be wrong and could cause these symptoms. Tell the patient the first two diagnoses on your differential list and the major tests you'd now like to perform.

Example: *"Ms. Swennis, Bobby has several aspects that might be causing him to have an increased temperature. As part of my investigation, I look for areas that might be infected and thus cause his body to react with a fever. Bobby has some redness of that left ear and some features that suggest a middle ear infection. These are things like redness and what appears to be fluid behind is eardrum on the left. By looking at it, his left ear really does look infected. Also, he has some swollen tonsils that also might be a source of infection. Either one or both of these may cause his other symptoms as well, like sore throat and decreased appetite. The first thing I'd like to do is obtain a swab of his throat to check for a common reason for a bacterial infection called "strep throat." Strep throat is caused by a bacteria called Streptococcus, which needs to be treated if present. It's not that treating this infection will make him feel significantly better, but rather it will prevent other rare complications of the infection, like heart or kidney problems. Also, since this is the flu season, I'd like to take another swab from his nose to test for the flu. It's an easy test but can more accurately test for this virus. As well, another aspect of investigating his fever is to obtain a little urine for analysis. Overall, I think Bobby will do fine, but I'd like to make sure with these tests. I'll be calling you in a few days with all the results so we may discuss them. Please excuse me while I step out to arrange these.*

Is there any other aspect of Bobby's healthcare we haven't already discussed? Ok then, thank you."

PATIENT NOTE

History: Include significant positives and negatives from history of present illness, past medical history, review of system(s), social history, and family history.

HPI: 9 y/o male with fever x 1 day. The mother states maximum witnessed temp to 102.3 occurred this A.M., which responded to acetaminophen. Recent onset cold symptoms x 2 wks with frequent exposure to cold weather. Symptom of sore throat, runny nose, and stuffy nose progressed to include decreased activity, decreased appetite, and subjective fever over the last day. Positive pain in left ear, mother denies discharge.

PMH: Prior otitis media while toddler.

PSH: Umbilical hernia repair.

Vaccinations up to date for age.

Tobacco: Mother denies exposure to smoke.

Meds: Acetaminophen x 2, last dose this A.M. Daily multivitamin.

FamH: Recent sick contacts, including mother, father, brother, sister.

Physical Examination: Indicate only pertinent positive and negative findings related to the patient's chief complaint.

VS Stable.

HEENT: Eyes: normal, PERLA. Left Ear: intact bulging TM, +erythema, +effusion. No discharge. Decreased mobility. Right Ear: normal appearing. Nose: normal. Throat: +post pharyngeal erythema, +symmetric tonsil swelling, +exudates. Uvula midline.

Neck: Mild anterior cervical lymphadenopathy. Neg Kernig's/Brudzinski's signs.

Lungs: Clear to auscultation bilaterally. No wheezes, rubs, or rhonchi.

Skin: No lesions, rashes, focal areas of erythema.

Differential Diagnosis: In order of likelihood (with 1 being the most likely), list up to 5 potential or possible diagnoses for this patient's presentation (in many cases, fewer than 5 diagnoses are likely)	Diagnostic Work-up: List immediate plans (up to 5) for further diagnostic work-up
1. Otitis media	1. Rapid antigen testing for strep throat
2. Viral pharyngitis	2. Influenza antigen testing.
3. Streptococcal pharyngitis	3. Urine analysis and culture
4. Bronchitis	4.
5. Cystitis	5.

1. Opening Scenario

Victoria Humsha, a 39-year-old female, has come to the physician's clinic for recent sleep problems.

2. Vital Signs

BP: 140/84 mmHg

Temp: 98.3° F (36.8° C)

HR: 66/minute, regular

RR: 16/minute

Weight: 188 lbs (85.3 kg)

Height: 5'0" (152 cm)

BMI: 36.7 kg/m²

3. Examinee Tasks

1. Obtain a focused history.

2. Perform a relevant physical examination. (Do not perform breast, pelvic/genital, or rectal examination.)

3. Discuss your initial diagnostic impression and your work-up plan.

4. After leaving the room, complete your patient note on the given form.

Are the Vital Signs Stable?

Subjective

Knock; enter. Introduce yourself, and place the first signpost.

"Hello, Ms. Humsha, I'm Dr. Hughman. I understand you've had some recent problems with sleep. Please tell me more about it."

"Hi, doc. I just **can't sleep**, that's all. I just can't sleep, and it's very hard on me. I've been to the doctor before, but he **just told me to 'tough it out,'** and he said it's because **I'm too fat**. He actually said that, he said, 'You're too fat.' So, needless to say, I switched doctors."

First indications of a difficult patient may be a story that appears very one-sided and unusual. Make sure not to respond with doubt or judgment to these initial indications.

An early signpost of what the patient can expect in the visit not only gives the patient an idea of what to expect but also allows the interview to be structured in a reasonable manner.

As the interview progresses, be on the lookout for personality traits such as "splitting," often seen in those with borderline personality disorder.

Splitting consists of demonizing some people in the patient's life while glorifying others. It's an outlook on relationships that sees others either as all enemy or all friend.

Technique for dealing with difficult patients:
Motivation—Name your motivation for questioning
Situation—Restate the patient coming to you for help
Empathy—Make a statement of empathy for the patient
Intentions—Signpost your intentions
Alternative—State clearly the alternative to continuing
Freedom—Remind them of their freedom to end the interview
Choice—Give them a final choice to continue

"Well, that sounds like a very bad experience. Please tell me more."

"So, now I still can't sleep and I feel too fat. I mean, I know I'm overweight but…anyway. So I'm here because I can't sleep. I haven't been able to in **months**. I just go to bed and **lay there and don't sleep**. It's like my body just feels so exhausted, but it's like I just can't sleep. My husband **sleeps like a log,** and I just lay there listening to his breathing."

"That's hard enough, too, it sounds like. Let me begin by asking a few questions about your sleep habits, and then we'll move on to a physical exam. Some blood work or other testing might be necessary and then I hope to find out what we can do. Is that alright?"

"Well, **that's what I'm here for**. I want you to do something. Just don't call me fat again."

"I will make sure to not call you any names at all. Can you tell me when you go to bed every night and when you wake up?"

"I go to bed at the normal time. Maybe **11:00 or midnight**. Then my kids have to get up for school at 6:30, and the lord knows my husband won't get them up, so **I have to.**"

"Ok. And you said you just lie there listening to your husband. Would you say, then, you have trouble falling asleep or staying asleep?"

"Obviously that means I can't fall asleep. I mean, I wouldn't just wake up and listen to him. I can't fall asleep for hours. I just lie there."

"Ok. Well, do you watch TV in bed or read at night when you can't fall asleep?"

"No, doctor, I just lie there. We've been over this. I just lie there, I just lie there!"

"Ma'am, I'm asking you these questions to clarify what your sleep habits are because you came in for me to evaluate your sleep problems. I think you've obviously had some frustration with prior attempts to get help as well as the frustration of living with your sleep issues. However, these questions are ones that help me understand what you're going through and are in no way intended to annoy you. I intend to ask further questions not only about your sleep but also about other aspects of your health. If you would not like to continue, you are free to end this appointment at any time. Otherwise, please expect further questions such as these. Would you like to continue?"

"Yeah, yeah, I'm just **tired**, like I said. I mean really tired. I've got a **headache**, too. I also have this disease, **fibromyalgia.** You should know what that is. So let's just do this appointment, and you can tell me what's wrong."

"Ok. Let's move on. Please tell me how much caffeine you drink during the day or night."

"I drink about **two cups of coffee** when I get up in the **morning**. I have maybe **one soda** during the day. That's it."

"Alright. Do you take any herbal or over-the-counter medicines?"

"**No**, I was on this stuff called **St. John's Wort,** but it didn't do anything at all. My friend, the healer, gave me it. Since then she was arrested for mail fraud. Anyway, it didn't work."

"How long has it been that you stopped taking that?"

"I don't know, whatever, a **few months** or so."

"Ok. How long exactly have you been having trouble sleeping?"

"Like, maybe **4 or 5 months**. I've never slept good but it's been probably that long since it became really bad."

"Have you taken any other medicines for sleep?"

"What? Like drugs? You think I'd do that? **No**. I don't take drugs. Thanks for asking."

"I don't mean drugs as in 'illegal drugs,' I mean medicines prescribed by a health-care provider."

"Yeah, I know what you mean. **No**, I said. I don't take drugs. I can't believe you asked me that!"

"Ma'am, again, these questions are not meant to offend in any way…"

"Yeah, they're just standard medical questions. Do you accuse everyone that comes in here of taking drugs?"

"Ma'am, again, you are free to end this appointment at any time if you wish. My questions relate to your health and health care and are not meant to offend you. The question I asked is 'Are there any medicines that you've taken for your sleep problems?'"

"**No**."

"Ok. Have you found anything else that might have been helpful, such as a glass of warm milk or showering before bed?"

"**No**, doctor. If I did, I wouldn't be here."

"Ok. How long does it take for you to fall asleep?"

"Like **2 hours** at least."

"Does your bed partner ever tell you that you snore or seem to stop breathing for moments during your sleep?"

"**No**, like I said earlier, he sleeps like a log. He wouldn't wake up if I had a seizure."

"Has anyone else ever told you that you snore?"

"[In a sarcastic tone] No, doctor, no one ever said I snore."

"Do you smoke or use tobacco?"

"**Yeah**, I smoke about a **pack a day**."

"How long have you done that?"

"All my life, like **20 years** I've smoked. It never had anything to do with my sleep."

"Ok. Would you like help quitting?"

"**Not at all**. I like to smoke."

"Do you drink alcohol?"

"**No**, not me. I'm not the drinker in the house."

"Does your husband drink excessively?"

"Are you kidding? He drinks like a fish. Every night."

A patient may mean to establish an unsaid respect for themselves by reacting to a certain line of questions. Don't be intimidated into not asking pertinent questions because the response may be to be offended. Reasonable health questions should never be construed as offensive by the patient.

"Does he ever get violent or verbally abusive when he drinks?"

"**Yeah**, he **yells a lot**. He can't do anything like hit me though. He knows I'd kill him."

"Do you feel safe in the home?"

"**Yeah**, he's just a jerk. He can't hurt me though."

"How about the children—does he ever yell or get violent with them?"

"Sometimes he **yells at them,** but he wouldn't dare hit them. He knows I'd put him on the ground."

"Would you like to talk to a counselor or abuse counselor about your home situation? Many people say that helps."

"**No**, no. I can handle him. We've been married for 22 years. I can handle him."

"Ok. I'd like to give you some resources to take home today in case his drinking ever turns abusive, ok? They have several phone numbers to people who will help if you need it."

"I **don't need** that crap but whatever gets you to move on."

"Have you ever felt depressed?"

"**Of course**, I've been depressed before. I live with a jerk, and my house is a wreck most of the time. That's what I took the Wort stuff for."

"Have you ever thought about killing yourself or hurting someone else?"

"**No**, not seriously. I'm not going to leave my family. I wouldn't do that."

"Have you had a decrease in appetite lately?"

"Oh, here we go again. I know I'm fat already. I eat too much, I know!"

Objections may be raised throughout the interview to personal questions. Revisit your motivation for asking the question.

"Ma'am a decreased appetite is a sign of depression that occurs in some people. Your personal weight has nothing to do with my question. I know these questions can be personal, but they give me a good picture of what might be going on. Have you had a decrease in appetite lately?"

"**No**, my appetite's fine."

"Do you have trouble looking forward to things the way you once did?"

"**Maybe**. I don't look forward to much."

"You also said you had a headache. Is that unusual for you?"

"I **get headaches almost every day**. My regular doctor says it goes with my fibromyalgia. I take aspirin for it."

"Does your fibromyalgia cause pain anywhere else?"

"Do you know what fibromyalgia is? Course it causes pain—my legs are hurting all the time."

"I do know what it is, ma'am, but I can't personally relate to the symptoms. Have you been on any medication for your fibromyalgia?"

"**No**, it was diagnosed by that same whacky doctor who told me I was too fat, so I never went back to him."

"Have you had any other problems such as nausea, vomiting, stomach pain, or diarrhea?"

"**No**, none of that."

"Have you ever had surgery for anything?"

"I had a **c-section** with my third child. He's 3 years old now."

"Ok. Do you have any allergies?"

"**No**."

"Has anyone in your family had similar problems as this?"

"Well, my **dad's dead** because he killed himself. I'm not upset about that though. He was a real jerk. My **mom** lives with my sister, and she just has **diabetes**."

"When was your father's suicide?"

"**Six months ago**. He did it in his car outside my mom's house. Can you believe that? He was such a crazy jerk!"

"That sounds very hard to deal with. Have you talked with a counselor or mental health-care worker about that?"

"**No**, not at all. Like I said, he was a jerk. Case closed, nothing more to say."

"Well sometimes, even though you may not want to think about things like that, it can help to talk about it. It may just help to go in and see if talking helps. Would you like me to put in a referral to a counselor?"

"**No**, I said I don't need it."

"Ok. Well, if you change your mind, please contact my office. I'll also write the number to a good counselor on the information I give you for your husband's alcohol problem, ok?"

"**Yeah**, whatever."

> If a patient seems to be distant and unwilling to explore an obviously emotionally traumatic event, offer them resources to get help after the visit. Don't get into a power struggle to force them into counseling.

Signpost for the Physical Exam

"Ok. I'd like to do a physical exam now, if you don't mind. Just let me **wash my hands**. It looks like your **vital signs** show some high blood pressure but are otherwise normal. Please let me first look in your eyes…"

Objective

Points for Every Exam:

- Wash hands.
- Comment on vital signs, even if normal.
- Tell the patient where you are going to examine and disrobe.
- Do not repeat painful maneuvers.

Physical Exam:

Perform a focused physical, by system, from the head down.

System	Exam elements	Findings in this patient
HEENT	Eyes: Exam pupils for light reactivity, unusual constriction, or unusual dilation. Throat: Use a light source such as an otoscope or penlight to examine the oral cavity and teeth. Examine the posterior pharynx and comment aloud on any abnormalities. Use a tongue depressor to gain a clear view if necessary. Ask the patient to say "Ah."	Eyes are PERRLA. Oral mucosa moist without obvious tooth breaks or decay. Pharynx is non-erythematous, uvula midline, no overt tonsillor hypertrophy, no exudates.
Thyroid	Observe the thyroid gland, and ask the patient to swallow before feeling the neck. Then, feel for the thyroid gland with both hands while standing behind the patient. Palpate the gland as the patient swallows again.	Normal, no enlargement

Continue to gather information as you do the physical exam. Ask about pertinent aspects of each system as you perform the exams. Comment aloud on any real or simulated abnormalities.

Example: *"Do you have trouble swallowing food or liquids?"*

Example: *"Have you recently had a sore throat or cold?"*

End of Case

End by explaining you have several ideas of what could be wrong and could cause these symptoms. Tell the patient the first two diagnoses on your differential list and the major tests you'd now like to perform.

Example: *"Ms. Humsha, there are several things that I think maybe contributing to your overall sleep problems. These are just possibilities, and some of the problems require more testing be done. One, however, might be your fibromyalgia. This disorder is sometimes linked to sleep problems and requires medications to reset your 'sleep timer.' That may be one area we explore in the future. As far as other medical problems, some people have a thyroid gland disorder that may cause sleep problems. That just means your thyroid gland may be producing too much or too little or too much hormone. It's a simple blood test to find that out. Also, a possible source of some of your daytime tiredness may be in something called 'obstructive sleep apnea.' That's a disorder people may get wherein they actually stop breathing at night just for a few seconds. What happens then is that their body stirs or wakes up just enough to start breathing again but not fully. People with this condition don't generally know they have it because they don't wake up fully but just enough to interrupt getting a full night's sleep. To evaluate you for this, I'd like to have you come into the hospital for an overnight stay that's monitored with certain machines and cameras. We can then tell if you wake up for these tiny periods during the night. Do you have any questions about that?"*

"No, I know what you mean. I can do that but not for a while. I'll have to check to see when I can do it."

"Ok. Also from our interview, I think you might have some other reasons in your life to have some depression or depression-related disorder. It sounds like your life is in a considerable amount of stress. I think anyone might have some trouble with the issues you're going through. For that, I'd encourage you to see a counselor. Sleep can be one of those areas that's very affected by your mood and stress level, so I wouldn't be surprised to find it has something to do with yours. I'd like to put in a referral for a mental health counselor for you, would you like that?"

"I...no, not right now."

"Ok. Well, please allow me to give you this information [handing the patient information sheets] about stress and resources for you to contact if you want to later. Please remember, my office is open during the day, or you can always go to the emergency room if you ever have a time that you or your kids don't feel safe in your home. Also, we are here to help so please come here or the ER if you need help with that, Ok? I'd like to step out now and arrange that blood work be done that I mentioned before.

Is there any other aspect of your health care we haven't already discussed? Ok then, thank you."

PATIENT NOTE

History

HPI: 39 y/o female presents with c/o daytime sleepiness and inability to fall asleep for 4-5 months. She describes several stressors, including possible depression, recent father's suicide, alcoholic and verbally abusive husband at home. She denies SI/HI. She states she has previous diagnosis of fibromyalgia, including accompanying daily headaches and leg pain. Question of previous w/u for possible OSA or obesity but patient states she didn't continue because of dislike of previous physician. Caffeine consumption 1-2 cups coffee and 1 soda per day. Pt smokes but denies interference with sleep. Denies alcohol use.

PMH: Fibromyalgia, headaches, historic sleep complaints.

PSH: Cesarean section—3 yrs ago.

Meds: Occasional aspirin.

FamH: Father—deceased, suicide 6 months ago.

Physical Exam

VS Stable, normal. Increased BP noted.

Psychiatric: Nondisheveled, Caucasian female appearing approximate stated age. Thought processes ordered and logical. Affect is euthymic and mood-appropriate but confrontational. No tangential or magical thinking. No delusions. Denies suicidal or homicidal ideation. Pt somewhat argumentative during interview.

HEENT: Eyes: PERRLA. Oral cavity: No visible abnormalities of the oral cavity or teeth. Throat: Normal, midline uvula, normal soft palate. No tonsillor hypertrophy, no tonsillor exudates. Neck: Supple.

Thyroid: No enlargement or abnormalities.

Differential Diagnosis: In order of likelihood (with 1 being the most likely), list up to 5 potential or possible diagnoses for this patient's presentation (in many cases, fewer than 5 diagnoses are likely)	Diagnostic Workup: List immediate plans (up to 5) for further diagnostic work-up
1. Fibromyalgia	1. TSH, free T4
2. Major depressive disorder	2. Overnight sleep study
3. Obstructive sleep apnea	3.
4. Thyroid dysfunction	4.
5. Bereavement	5.

---

1. Opening Scenario

Vince Casner, a 49-year-old male, has come to the emergency department for back pain.

2. Vital Signs

BP: 130/82 mmHg

Temp: 98.6° F (37.0° C)

HR: 62/minute, regular

RR: 12/minute

3. Examinee Tasks

1. Obtain a focused history.

2. Perform a relevant physical examination. (Do not perform breast, pelvic/genital, or rectal examination.)

3. Discuss your initial diagnostic impression and your work-up plan.

4. After leaving the room, complete your patient note on the given form.

Are the Vital Signs Stable?

Subjective

Knock; enter. Introduce yourself, and place the first signpost.

"Hello Mr. Casner, I'm Dr. Morgan. I understand you've been having some back pain lately. Please tell me more about it."

"Yeah, doc. My back is just killing me. I **threw it out again**. This happens every month or two, and I just can't move. I usually see my normal doctor about this, but he won't be open until Monday. This one's a real killer, too. I can **hardly move**."

"It does look like you're in pain. When did you do this?"

"**Yesterday**. I'm a foreman for J & T Construction, and I was **lifting** some couplings yesterday and lifted them about this high [indicating about 3 feet off the ground], and I **just froze**. I just couldn't move and knew I threw it out again. I knew when I did it, and all I could do is freeze, like this [showing the position he was in]. So, yesterday was Friday, and I took some **Tylenol** like my doctor says, but I just can't make it. So I came in."

"Ok. I know hurting your back can be very painful. How long have you had this problem?"

"Oh, hell, it started happening maybe **10 years ago**. I don't usually say anything. I **don't like to come to the doctor**, you know. I'm just not one to come in unless I really hurt myself, I just don't believe in it. I'll just sit there and take the pain usually. You all have better things to do than deal with my old back. I only do this about once every month or two. My doctor usually just **gives me some pills** and sends me home. I don't like taking anything, but I just go to bed and it usually helps."

"Have you ever had any X-rays or other tests done on your back?"

"Yeah, I got **X-rays** and a **CT** and an **MRI** done when I left Kansas City about **9 months ago**. I'm real jacked up! The MRI showed a slipped disc at two levels, not one, and something they called degeneration of the discs between most of the bones in my lower back. They said 'I can't believe you're still working.' It don't slow me down though. I have a really, really **high tolerance for pain**."

"Does this pain radiate down your legs or into other parts of your back?"

"Sometimes it hurts in my **right leg**."

"Have you had any problems moving that leg?"

"**Yeah**, sometimes, now that you mention it."

"When does that happen?"

"Umm, it happened **last week**, I couldn't move it for a minute or two. I was eating lunch and went to get up, and it **didn't work quite right**, you know?"

"Did you fall when you tried to walk?"

"**No**, I could feel, like, I couldn't move it, so I didn't walk right away. After a minute it worked."

"Did you have any back pain at the time?"

"**No**, I just hurt my back yesterday."

"Have you had problems moving your legs since this injury or back pain?"

"**No**, not this time."

"Alright. Can you describe the pain for me?"

"It hurts on both sides, you know, and it goes down the back of my leg. Down to about here [indicating the middle posterior thigh]."

"Ok. Have you had a fever since you hurt your back?"

"**Yeah**, I think so."

"How high was your temperature?"

"Well, I didn't take it, but **I felt like it**, you know? Like, I felt like I had a fever or something."

"Was that after or before your injury?"

"It was, umm, **after**."

"Ok. On a scale of 0 to 10, 10 being the worst pain imaginable, where would you rate your pain right now?"

Look for clues to the patient's agenda. Alluding to the treatment they want is a clue that the patient is suggesting a desired course of action.

Don't make decisions on work-up or management based on results a patient reports to you of prior tests. Either research their results or obtain new testing.

Be on the lookout for incongruencies of symptoms relating to time, duration, severity, and accompanying symptoms.

"I'd say an **11**, doc. I mean it really hurts, and I've got that real **high tolerance for pain**. This one really hurts; my other doc would just **give me some medicine** and send me to bed."

"Ok. Have you taken anything for your pain since it happened?"

"**No**, I try not to take anything because of my pain tolerance. I mean, I did take some Tylenol, but that was it. It hasn't helped."

"Are you on any other medications?"

"I'm on a blood pressure medicine called **atenolol** right now. I've tried them all for this pain. I just need some time to work it through."

"Ok. What medicines have you tried for the back pain?"

"**You name it**, doc. I've tried **everything over-the-counter** like **Motrin** and stuff. My doctor gave me stuff like **gabapentin** and **lyrica** and **tramadol**. He tried muscle relaxers like **cyclobenzaprine** and a bunch of others. He gave me **shots** before for the pain. I can't take stuff like **hydrocodone** because that makes me sick; I **threw up** 10 times once when he gave me that. The only thing he gave me that helped was this little pink pill. I can't remember the name…it was pamicet or namicet or something."

"Was it called Percocet?"

"**Yeah**, that's it. I hate to take that stuff at all, but that's the only thing that works. I don't like medicines, doc. I can't stand taking stuff. I'm the kind of guy that just toughs things out; I hate medicine. But that's all that's ever even touched the pain is Percocet. I know because I've tried it all."

"Have you tried toradol? It's a shot given in your muscle or through an IV?"

"**Yeah**, I tried that—doesn't touch it."

"Have you ever been seen by an orthopedic surgeon?"

"**Nah**, I got a referral in Kansas City but then had to move. My doctor here said he's going to refer me. He said the next time I come in he was going to take care of that."

"Have you ever gotten a shot in the back such as steroids?"

"I **tried that, too**. That's how bad my back is. It just didn't help, though. If I just sleep it off, I'm fine in a few days."

"Ok. You said earlier you had some high blood pressure. Is there anything else in your past medical history?"

"**No**, that's it. Like I said, I'm a healthy guy. I do a lot for my work and don't like to go to doctors unless I really need it, you know?"

"Yeah, I can understand that. Have you ever had any surgeries?"

"I had my **wisdom teeth** pulled out when I was a kid but **otherwise no**. I don't like surgeons more than I don't like needles."

"How about allergies? Do you have any allergies to anything?"

"**Nope**, well, maybe that hydrocodone. I threw up when I took it."

"Well, that actually doesn't sound like a usual allergy but more of a side effect that can happen in some people. But, nonetheless, we'll stay away from that. Are you on anything else other than the atenolol?"

A technique of some drug-seeking patients is to get the physician to name the drug they're seeking. This technique sometimes helps the physician to think it was their own idea for the medication, not the patient's. However, the patient will often state that only that medicine will work for them.

Another popular technique of patients seeking drugs is repeatedly trying to convince the physician they don't like to take medicines. However, they'll also frame the situation as the medicine they want is the only one that works, despite them not wanting it. This technique aims at building trust with the physician.

In dealing with a possible drug-seeking patient, it's important to not promise a particular type of treatment. Don't give clues or hints that you will follow the course of action they're suggesting.

"Nothing."

"Have there been any similar problems in your family?"

"No, my **family's healthy**. They keep wondering why I'm coming to the doctor as much as I am. They stand clear of you guys."

"How about tobacco—do you use it at all?"

"**Nah**, I used to smoke, but I quit 10 years ago. I had enough of it and just stopped altogether."

"Great, that's hard to do. How about drinking?"

"I have a **beer or two when I watch football** during the season. I don't drink regularly, though."

Signpost for the Physical Exam

"Ok. I'd like to do a physical exam now, if you don't mind. Just let me **wash my hands**. It looks like your **vital signs** are normal. Please let me look at your back…"

Objective

Points for Every Exam:

- Wash hands.
- Comment on vital signs, even if normal.
- Tell the patient where you are going to examine and disrobe.
- Do not repeat painful maneuvers.

Physical Exam:

Perform a focused physical, by system, from the head down.

System	Exam elements	Findings in this patient
Back	Ask the patient to disrobe and observe the back for erythema, swelling, deformity, or spasm in the upright and sitting positions. Ask him to point to the maximum area of pain; avoid that area at first, then palpate it last. Note the ischial spine relative heights. Complete ROM maneuvers, including flexion, extension, lateral, and rotation, communicating with the patient to determine the most painful maneuvers or radiation of pain. Complete ipsilateral and contralateral leg raise testing and FABER testing.	The patient points to approximately the L4 level, stating pain is bilateral. Palpation of midline spinous processes in the lumbar area does not produce tenderness. Much perispinal tenderness is found in this general area. Flexion/extension is not limited by pain. Rotation and lateral ROM normal on each side. Ischial spine heights are approximately equal. The patient does complain of pain in the right leg on the supine ipsilateral straight leg test, which is not found on the sitting straight leg raise. Negative FABER test, bilaterally. Axial loading test positive for lower back pain.
Neurologic	Perform tactile sense testing of the lower extremities as well as checking for proprioception and sharp/dull testing. Assess deep tendon reflexes and motor strength. Observe his gait including heel- and toe-walks. Rectal tone is not indicated in this patient.	Normal tactile sense of bilateral lower extremities including sharp/dull. Normal proprioception and deep tendon reflexes. Somewhat impaired gait because of pain, but normal heel-/toe-walking.

Continue to gather information as you do the physical exam. Ask about pertinent aspects of each system as you perform the exams. Comment aloud on any real or simulated abnormalities.

Example: *"Do you have any numbness or tingling down here [indicating his toes and feet]?"*

Example: *"Have you had trouble walking since you injured your back?"*

End of Case

End by explaining you have several ideas of what could be wrong and could cause these symptoms. Tell the patient the first two diagnoses on your differential list and the major tests you'd now like to perform.

Example: *"Mr. Casner, there are several possibilities that might be at the root of your back pain. The cause of back pain itself can be very hard to pinpoint. That goes for your kind of pain as well, when it comes on all of a sudden and is as severe as you describe. The most common cause of pain like yours is a spasm of the back muscles themselves. Back muscles, called postural muscles, are not only under our conscious control—they're also controlled by our higher brain functions to help us stand up. That means we don't have to constantly think about keeping ourselves upright when we stand but that our brain controls it without us thinking about it. But the downside to that is that sometimes our back muscles spasm outside of our control, and sometimes that can be very painful. Another possibility is that you did do some structural damage to one of the discs in between the vertebrae of the bones. Because you've had some radiating pain into your leg, I'd like to take some X-rays of your back to find out if the spaces between the vertebrae look right or not. A disc in your back may either bulge out of position or rupture out of position, both of which can cause pressure on the nearby exiting nerves and cause symptoms of pain down the legs or into other areas. But, keep in mind, a plain X-ray is not the best test to evaluate if this or other problems have occurred that deal with the nerves. However, it's the best test to do here in the ER to determine if there are serious problems with the bones or spaces between the bones in your back. If I don't see anything on the X-ray, there is the possibility you still might need an MRI, although that should be ordered and explored by your primary care physician. This X-ray will also be able to tell me if, for some reason, you had a fracture of a vertebral bone that might be the cause of these symptoms. I'd like to step out now and order this X-ray with my nurse. Afterward, expect to come back to this room until the results are ready. When they are, I'll come right back in to discuss them with you.*

Is there any other aspect of your health care we haven't already discussed? Ok then, thank you."

PATIENT NOTE

History: Include significant positives and negatives from history of present illness, past medical history, review of system(s), social history, and family history.

HPI: 49 y/o male c/o back pain x approx 24 hours. He states pain is 11/10 and came on when lifting heavy objects during work. Pain caused him to freeze position at onset and has reportedly restricted normal movement since. He states pain is in lumbar area and radiates down right leg to approximately mid-posterior thigh. One reported episode of motor disturbance 1 week ago although unrelated to back pain or injury. Patient is able to ambulate and has self-medicated only with acetaminophen. History includes reported w/u and episodes treated by regular physician with Percocet. Reported prior testing includes MRI but results not available today. Pt states other medications such as OTC NSAIDs, toradol, hydrocodone are ineffective or cause vomiting, thus requests Percocet to treat pain until he is able to contact regular physician in 2 days.

Meds: Atenolol.

PMH: Previous episodes of functional back pain.

PSH: Wisdom tooth extraction.

Smoke: Denies.

Drink: Denies.

FamH: Noncontributory.

Physical Exam: Indicate only pertinent positive and negative findings related to the patient's chief complaint.

VS Stable, normal.

Back: No midline ttp. Moderate perispinal ttp. ROM normal, including flexion/extension, rotation, lateral bending. Ischial spine heights are approximately equal. Supine right ipsilateral straight leg raise positive, finding not found on sitting straight leg raise. Negative FABER test, bilaterally. Axial loading test positive for lower back pain.

Neurologic: Normal sharp/dull and tactile sense of lower extremities. Normal proprioception and deep tendon reflexes. Somewhat impaired gait resulting from pain but normal heel-/toe-walking.

Differential Diagnosis: In order of likelihood (with 1 being the most likely), list up to 5 potential or possible diagnoses for this patient's presentation (in many cases, fewer than 5 diagnoses are likely)	Diagnostic Workup: List immediate plans (up to 5) for further diagnostic work-up
1. Drug-seeking behavior	1. Lumbar X-rays
2. Malingering	2.
3. Muscular back spasm	3.
4. Bulging intervertebral disc	4.
5. Ruptured intervertebral disc	5.

35   Difficult Patient: Non-English Speaking

1. Opening Scenario

Abbas Muhumudi, a 54-year-old Arabic language-speaking male, comes to the clinic complaining of heartburn-type pain.

2. Vital Signs

BP: 132/84 mmHg

Temp: 98.7° F (37.1° C)

HR: 70/minute, regular

RR: 12/minute

3. Examinee Tasks

1. Obtain a focused history.

2. Perform a relevant physical examination. (Do not perform breast, pelvic/genital, or rectal examination.)

3. Discuss your initial diagnostic impression and your work-up plan.

4. After leaving the room, complete your patient note on the given form.

It's important to establish the ground rules with the translator before the interview. Have the translator speak as if they were the patient and translate your words to the patient in the same manner. Thus, dialogue is between the patient and doctor through the translator, instead of the translator having two simultaneous conversations.

Are the Vital Signs Stable?

Subjective

Knock; enter. Introduce yourself, and place the first signpost.

Note the presence of a translator.

"Hello, Mr. Muhumudi, I'm Dr. Jones."

Translator: "Hello doctor, I'm Chidell. **I'm the translator** for the hospital for Arabic languages. I'm here to translate for you with Mr. Muhumudi. Please use me for speaking to Mr. Muhumudi."

"Ok. Nice to meet you Mr. Chidell. That's fine with me. [Nod acknowledgement to the patient and make eye contact.] Thanks for your help.

[Addressing the patient] *Hello, Mr. Muhumudi, I'm Dr. Jones. How may I help you today?"*

[Arabic dialogue] "He says, doctor, he is here because of his heartburn. He says he would like to know if he can get help with the pain in his stomach."

"Well, ok. Mr. Chidell, please translate my words to him directly as best as possible. Then please tell me what he's saying using his words. Please tell me as directly as possible what he's saying, ok? That helps me to more accurately understand him so I can use you to, sort of, talk to him, if you know what I mean.

Mr. Muhumudi, can you describe the pain for me?"

"**Sure**, doctor. No problem. I'll try to **translate as directly as I can**.

[Arabic dialogue] I have some **pain in my stomach** right here [indicating his **epigastric area**]. It hurts me when I eat a **big meal,** and it hurts me at **night**. It's, like, a **sharp pain** right in the center, and it comes on **every single day**."

"Ok. Does it start in your stomach and radiate anywhere?"

[Arabic dialogue] "It starts here [indicating his epigastric area] and **goes up** like this [indicating radiation to his chest]. I **cannot control it,** and it seems like I am in pain sometimes, much."

"I'm sorry to hear that. I will try to do what I can for you to figure out what this pain is. I will have to ask you some questions and maybe need to do some tests." [pause for translation]

"I will have to do a physical exam on you before you leave, and I hope to be able to tell better what this might be. Ok?"

[Arabic dialogue] "**Ok**. I hope you can help because it hurts at **night mostly**."

"Ok. I understand it is mostly at night. Can you tell me more specifically when it happens at night?"

[Arabic dialogue] "Yes, it happens **when I eat and lie down to sleep**. I feel like it hurts most then. I can sometimes feel it when I am **finished eating lunch**. It hurts me **after I eat**, mostly, too."

"Would you describe the pain as burning or sharp or dull; how would you describe it?"

[Arabic dialogue] "I say it feels **burning but sharp** right here [indicating epigastric region]."

"On a scale of 0 to 10, 10 being the worst pain imaginable, how high would you rate this pain?"

[Arabic dialogue] "I would say it is **8**. It makes it **difficult to sleep** sometimes and makes me **not want to eat food**."

"Ok. How long have you had this problem?"

[Arabic dialogue] "I've had this for **at least 2 years**, maybe longer. I don't know. I feel like it has caused problems since my **daughter got married and left the house**. I say she did this to me [in a humorous tone]."

"Ok. Sometimes it's hard to see one's child move away, isn't it? Did it come on right away, or did it take some time?"

No matter what language the patient speaks, think about each answer and interpret minor differences in speech.

If you have been given information you think may be inaccurate because of translation, try to repeat the same question using different language.

Be sensitive to cues of cultural values that may not be customary in the United States but may indicate great importance in the patient's native culture.

[Arabic dialogue] "It **took a while**. It didn't come on right away. Maybe it started a few nights per week. Then it happened more and more, and now it happens all the time."

"Do you have other symptoms, such as vomiting or pain when you swallow food?"

[Arabic dialogue] "**No**. I have a good time eating. I **like to eat,** but it is just some foods that I get this pain. But most foods I get this pain with. I don't vomit with eating."

"What foods seem to cause this pain?"

[Arabic dialogue] "Maybe if I eat **spices** or things that have **much fat** in them, maybe, then I get this pain. It is not with foods that are simple. Bread and cheese I do not get this pain with."

"When you're eating, do you feel full before you think you should or before you used to feel full?"

[Arabic dialogue] "**Sometimes**. I eat **beef and chicken** sometimes, and I used to eat more. I eat less now because I'm full now. This is not a big problem. I eat enough."

"Does this pain come on more when you lie down or when you are standing or sitting?"

[Arabic dialogue] "It **does not matter**; when I sit **after evening meal**, it comes on, too. But especially if I **lie down** or if I have meal late and go to bed."

"Ok. Have you tried anything for this problem?"

[Arabic dialogue] "I have tried to take some **blue pills** before, but they do not work. My doctor back home gave them to me. I don't know the name of them."

"It's very hard for me to know what those are. Are you still taking them?"

[Arabic dialogue] "No. I stopped because they **don't help me**. That's why I come here for you to help me."

"I understand. Ok. Are you taking any other medications?"

[Arabic dialogue] "I am also taking other medicines from my doctor back home. It is **hydrocholorthiazide** from him; it is also **aspirin**. He says they are for my **blood pressure** and my **blood**."

"Ok. Do you take any other medicines or treatments such as teas or certain foods meant to heal?"

[Arabic dialogue] "**No**, I don't take tea for medicine. I take tea everyday for drinking, but it is chai; it is what we do."

"I understand. But do you have any other treatment you have done?"

[Arabic dialogue] "**No**, no."

"I understand you have high blood pressure. Do you have any other problems with your health?"

[Arabic dialogue] "My doctor, at home, said I should take **aspirin** every day. He said for my blood. I don't have anything else wrong with me. Just my pain in my stomach."

Never criticize a fellow health-care worker in another culture. It not only crosses cultural barriers but is very unprofessional.

Asking about other cultural treatments is very important.

"Have you had any surgeries?"

[Arabic dialogue] "**No**, none."

"How much tea do you drink?"

[Arabic dialogue] "It is not much. I drink **tea in the morning and in the afternoon**. I **don't drink coffee** like in the U.S. I drink tea, you see. Maybe, umm...**two or three cups** is all."

"Ok. Do you use tobacco at all?"

[Arabic dialogue] "I **smoke,** but everybody smokes. I smoke maybe **20 cigarettes a day** or so. Not a problem."

"Ok. How long have you smoked that much?"

[Arabic dialogue] "I smoke that much all my life. Maybe **since age 10**. My doctor says it is good to smoke some. Everyone smokes."

"Alright. In medicine, we have found this to be very bad for your health. Would you like to quit smoking? Would you like me to help you quit smoking—to make it easier?"

[Arabic dialogue] "**No**. I like it, and everyone in my family smokes."

"Ok. Do you drink alcohol at all?"

[Arabic dialogue] "I do not drink alcohol."

"Alright. Do you have any allergies to anything?"

[Arabic dialogue] "**No**, no. I'm not allergic to anything."

"Is anyone in your family sick, or have they been sick lately? That is, are there any diseases that run in your family?"

[Arabic dialogue] "**No**, nothing."

> Be open-minded to differences in cultural health. Many cultures regard tobacco as unrelated to health.

Signpost for the Physical Exam

"Ok. Mr Muhumudi, I'd like to do a physical exam now, if you don't mind. Just let me wash my hands. It looks like your **vital signs are normal,** so please allow me to listen to your chest..."

> A note on time: For this type of interview, time during the interview phase may last too long for a complete history. Thus, if using a translator, try to combine the interview and physical exams.

Objective

Points for Every Exam:

- Wash hands.
- Comment on vital signs, even if normal.
- Tell the patient where you are going to examine and disrobe.
- Do not repeat painful maneuvers.

Physical Exam:

Perform a focused physical, by system, from the head down.

System	Exam elements	Findings in this patient
Heart	Listen for heart sounds in at least 4 different auscultation points. Feel for PMI. While auscltating the heart, feel radial and peripheral pulses. Check capillary refill.	RRR, no murmurs/rubs/gallops. Peripheral pulses 2+ bilaterally. Cap refill <2 secs.
Lungs	Auscultate the posterior lung fields. Make sure to listen to 6 points on the posterior lung fields.	Clear to auscultation bilaterally
Abdomen	Listen for bowel sounds. Ask the patient where the pain has historically been. Gently palpate all 4 quadrants and the epigastrim, palpating the most painful area last. Check Murphy's sign. Check for rebound tenderness over McBurney's point.	Normal BS's, no bruit's. No ttp, including over the epigastrim. No masses.

Continue to gather information as you do the physical exam. Comment aloud on any real or simulated abnormalities.

Example: *"Does it hurt more in this area?* [indicating the epigastrum]*"*

Example: *"Can you show me what position makes this pain worse?"*

End of Case

End by explaining you have several ideas of what could be wrong and could cause these symptoms. Tell the patient the first two diagnoses on your differential list and the major tests you'd now like to perform.

Example: *"Mr. Muhumudi, there are several health-related problems that may be causing the pain in your abdomen and stomach. The most likely problem is something called reflux disease. Reflux is basically acid in the stomach that abnormally travels up into the esophagus, the tube between your mouth and stomach, and burns the lining of the tube.*

[pause for translation] *This acid should remain in the stomach, but instead it travels upward. This happens sometimes for several reasons but most commonly because the muscle at the top of the stomach opens more than it should. That is the most likely cause of your pain.*

[pause for translation] *However, there are other possibilities as well. Your pain might be caused by an ulcer in your stomach or intestine. This can cause pain that hurts more when you eat foods that are spicy. It is hard to tell if there is an ulcer there, but the best way is to look at the stomach with a tiny camera.*

[pause for translation] *This camera is on the end of a long tube that is placed down your throat during a procedure. I would like to have you complete this procedure to evaluate for this possibility. The tube can also take samples, or biopsies, of the stomach lining if we need to. That can help us make sure there aren't other possibilities, such as cancer.*

[pause for translation] *I think cancer would be unusual in your case, but we can't tell unless we are able to look with a camera and take samples if we need to.*

[pause for translation] *There are other tests I would also like to obtain on you, including blood tests and a test that evaluates the air you exhale. These tests can also tell me information that can indicate what might be causing your pain.*

[pause for translation] *I would like to get the blood and breath tests today if we can. I would also like to make an appointment for you to come back for the test to have the scope done, ok?* [pause for translation]

[Arabic dialogue] *"Yes doctor. I understand."*

"The test with the scope will take place in this office, and you can go home after the procedure. You will be given medicines to make you very sleepy during the procedure but you will be, sort of, half-asleep. Not fully asleep.

[pause for translation]*During the procedure, you should be able to follow our directions, but you may not remember it when you wake up, ok? When you come back, you should consider this procedure to take all day, though, ok?* [pause for translation]

However, it is not a surgery. Just a way to look at the lining of your stomach.

Do you have any questions about this?" [pause for translation]

[Arabic dialogue] No, doctor. I understand."

"Do you have any questions at all for me?"

[Arabic dialogue] *"No, doctor, this is fine."*

"Ok. I will step out now and have my nurse return to arrange for the testing and the best time to perform the procedure. After all the testing has been done, I would like to see you back to discuss it. Thank you." [pause for translation]

PATIENT NOTE

History: Include significant positives and negatives from history of present illness, past medical history, review of system(s), social history, and family history.

HPI: 54 y/o male with chief complaint of pain in the epigastric region associated with lying down after eating. Interview conducted through translator. Pt c/o sharp/ burning sensation in epigastrum that radiates into chest made worse by spicy food and sitting or laying position after eating. Pain comes on almost every night for the last 2 years after a gradual onset. + early satiety with meat containing meals. He denies nausea/vomiting/dysphagia.

Meds: Aspirin and hydrochlorothiazide.

PMH: Hypertension.

PSH: None.

Tobacco: 1ppd × 44 years.

Alcohol use: Denies.

FamH: Noncontributory.

Physical Exam: Indicate only pertinent positive and negative findings related to the patient's chief complaint.

VS Stable, normal.

Heart: RRR no murmurs, rubs, or gallops. Peripheral pulses 2+ bilaterally. Normal cap refill.

Lung: Clear to auscultation bilaterally. No wheezes, rhonchi, or rales.

Abdomen: Normal BSs, no bruit's. No ttp, including over the epigastrim. No hepatosplenomegally. No masses. No peritoneal signs.

Differential Diagnosis: In order of likelihood (with 1 being the most likely), list up to 5 potential or possible diagnoses for this patient's presentation (in many cases, fewer than 5 diagnoses are likely)	Diagnostic Workup: List immediate plans (up to 5) for further diagnostic work-up.
1. Gastroesophageal reflux disease	1. Urea breath test (*H. pylori* breath test)
2. Chronic gastritis	2. CBC with differential
3. Peptic ulcer disease	3. Amylase/Lipase
4. Pancreatitis	4. Esophagogastroduodenoscopy (EGD)
5. Stomach malignancy	5.

1. Opening Scenario

Andy Lightfoot, a 22-year-old male, called the clinic office with complaints of abdominal pain.

2. Vital Signs

None reported.

3. Examinee Tasks

1. Obtain a focused history.

2. Do not perform a physical examination and leave that portion blank on the patient note.

3. Discuss your initial diagnostic impression and your work-up plan.

4. After leaving the room, complete your patient note on the given form.
Press the speaker button on the phone to be connected with the caller.

Introduce yourself, and place the first signpost.

Don't take any expressions the patient says literally.

"Hello Mr. Lightfoot, this is Dr. Franks. How may I help you this afternoon?"

"Hi Dr. Franks, it's Andy Lightfoot. I'm having a lot of **pain** right now. My **stomach's** killing me, and it feels like my insides are about to explode!"

"Alright, Andy. How long have you felt like this?"

"It's been about **4 hours**. I was alright before I got up to go to work. I ate **breakfast,** and then the pain started. It feels like someone's **jabbing me with a knife** inside. It hurts really bad. I **threw up**, like, **five times** already this morning. I wouldn't have called if it wasn't so bad. I'm sorry I couldn't make an appointment."

"That's ok, Andy. I know it's not easy to make appointments sometimes when you have immediate problems. Let me ask some questions about this pain, and we'll figure out what to do. You said it feels like someone's stabbing you from the inside. Where does it hurt?"

Often when a patient says "stomach," they mean abdomen. Thus, don't take patients' anatomical descriptions literally.

"It hurts in my **stomach,** sort of. I mean, it hurts right at the **top** of my belly."

"Does that mean it doesn't hurt in the lower part or on the sides?"

"**No**, kind of in the top."

"Ok. Does the pain radiate anywhere, like into your back or shoulder?"

"**Yeah**, my **back hurts**, too. I didn't notice that until this thing started. It might be because I've had problems with it in the past. It hurts in the **middle** right now, though."

"How long has your back hurt like this?"

"Maybe the same time as this belly pain. I don't know. I have lower back pain all the time, though. It just doesn't feel like this."

"Ok. Has the location of the abdominal pain changed since it started?"

"**No**, not really. It's been right there. It seems like its **getting worse**."

"Have you had this kind of pain before?"

"I've had **stomach problems**. I was put on a medicine for it, but it's never been this bad."

"Have you ever had an episode like this?"

"I don't know. The last time I had a bunch of pain like this was, like, **6 months ago**. I was able to just sleep it off with some **pain medicines** my sister gave me."

"Do you remember what those pills were?"

"**No**, not really. I never knew."

"Ok. You said you were prescribed some medicine—what medicine is that?"

"It's called **omeprazole**. It hasn't helped a whole lot, so I **stopped taking it** a **week ago**. I ran out and just didn't get the refill."

"Ok. When you feel this pain, is it constant, or does it come and go?"

"It's **always there**. Maybe worse a little bit at times, but it feels pretty constant."

"You said you vomited earlier; was there any blood in that?"

"**No**, not really. It was just the eggs and pancakes I had for breakfast."

"Ok. It sounds like you were able to eat, then. Did you eat before or after the pain started?"

"It was before. I couldn't eat afterward."

"Did you eat anything other than the eggs and pancakes?"

"I had some milk, too. And a little yogurt. I don't know. It wasn't anything real unusual. My girlfriend makes me this kind of thing about twice a week. I normally eat a **big breakfast** then **skip lunch** because I'm in class."

"Alright, on a scale of 0 to 10, 10 being the worst pain imaginable, where would you rate this pain?"

"It's a **10**, at least a 10."

"I'm sorry to hear that. It must be very hard to take. So you had this pain first start when you were eating, huh?"

"**Yeah**, at least that's when it started. I went to class, and it just got **worse and worse**."

"How quick did it get worse—over minutes or hours?"

When a patient confesses to taking another patient's pain medications, don't admonish them for this because that will only make them hesitant to talk about other points they think you might frown on.

Transition statement of empathy.

"I'd say it took **about an hour** to get bad. Once it started, it kept getting worse. I threw up once in the school bathroom then came home and did some more. What do you think it is?"

"Well, I can't tell just yet. I'm going to ask a few more questions and determine if you should come in to the clinic or emergency room or see if we can have you stay home. I can't tell as much over the phone, though, because you're not here for me to examine. Nonetheless, we'll be able to talk and figure out what to do, ok?"

"Ok."

"Have you had any diarrhea with this?"

"**No**, I haven't gone to the bathroom at all. I did pee a little but **nothing else**."

"Ok. Have you felt hot at all, like you might have a fever?"

"**No**, not really."

"Have you had any problems breathing?"

"**No**, not really. It **hurts my stomach if I take a deep breath**."

"Ok. How about pain in your chest?"

"**No**, none of that."

"Any problems with lightheadedness?"

"**No**."

"Ok. I understand you've been to the doctor for that medication, omeprazole. Have you seen them for this type of pain or other stomach problems in the past?"

"I got that medicine, and that was supposed to help my stomach. It didn't really, and that's why I didn't refill it. He said it was **reflux** or something—**acid reflux**, I think. That's all I've seen him for."

"Ok. How about other things you've seen the doctor for? Have you ever spent the night in the hospital?"

"**No**, I've never spent the night. I have **eczema**, too, but that hasn't flared up in about a year. Nothing else."

"Have you ever had a surgery?"

"No."

"Has anyone in your family had any major illnesses, especially anything like this?"

"**No**, my dad had a shoulder operation last year but nothing else."

"Ok. Do you drink alcohol?"

"**Yeah**, sometimes."

"How much do you drink?"

Judge if the CAGE questions will add anything to the encounter.

"Maybe about a **beer every night**. **More on the weekends** when I go out."

"When was the last time you drank?"

"**Last night**, a buddy of mine had a party. It was a **few beers and a shot**, though. I didn't get drunk or anything."

"Have you ever noticed pain in your abdomen or stomach after or when you drink alcohol?"

"Nope. Like I said, I didn't have that much."

"Let me just ask a few more questions about your alcohol consumption. I'm asking to try to determine if you drink enough for it to be related to this pain. Have you ever tried to cut down on the amount of alcohol you take in?"

"No, not really."

"Have you ever felt annoyed by anyone bringing up how much you drink?"

"Heck no. Most people I know drink much more than I do."

"Have you ever felt guilty because of your drinking?"

"No."

"Have you ever had an 'eye opener,' or a drink in the morning to help get you going?"

"No way."

"Ok. How about other things, such as tobacco products? Do you use any of them?"

"I dip when I go out sometimes. I haven't done that in a while though. I don't smoke."

End of Case

End by explaining you have several ideas of what could be wrong and could cause these symptoms. Make sure to recommend either for or against coming to the clinic/hospital and in what timeframe. Tell the patient the first few diagnoses on your differential list and the major tests you'd now like to perform.

Example: *"Andy, after listening to your symptoms, I think it's best you come in to the emergency room to be seen. The fact that you're having an unusually severe bought of pain along with the history of treating stomach problems concerns me for an ulcer or a serious consequence of an ulcer, where there is actually a hole formed in the stomach or intestine. That can be life-threatening, and over the phone, I'm not able to make a complete assessment or order the necessary tests to make sure this is not happening. When you come in, the emergency physician will be able to better determine what is causing your pain if it isn't actually an ulcer. If it's not, there are several other possibilities, from just gas pains to other diseases such as problems with your pancreas. These do, however, need to be evaluated right away because your pain is so severe. Do you think you can come in for me?"*

"Yeah, I think so."

"Ok, good. I'll call the emergency room and make sure they're aware of what we talked about and your case. I can't say how long it will take to see a doctor, but they'll at least know you're coming. Do you have a ride to the hospital?"

"Yeah, I can get one."

"Ok, good. I'm going to let you go arrange a ride. If you aren't able to, please call back and we'll arrange an ambulance to come get you. Do you have any questions? Ok, then thanks very much, and we'll talk soon."

PATIENT NOTE

History: Include significant positives and negatives from history of present illness, past medical history, review of system(s), social history, and family history.

HPI: 22 y/o male with severe abdominal pain x 4 hours. Pain began after heavy meal and over the course of about 1 hour built to 10/10 pain. Accompanying symptoms include nausea/vomiting and pain radiating to the midback. Prior evaluation by regular physician produced prescription for omeprazole, which the patient tried then chose not refill the prescription because of ineffect. No medicine x 1 wk. Prior self-treatment of similar episode with unknown pain med 6 months ago. Denies diarrhea, chest pain, respiratory complaints (although deep inhalation causes worsening of pain), lightheadedness, or subjective fever. Pain stated to be grossly unrelated to alcohol consumption although last drink the night before pain started.

PMH: Question of GERD vs PUD, Eczema.

PSH: None.

Tobacco: Denies.

Alcohol use: Approx 1 beer/night. Increased social drinking on weekends. Last drink: the night before symptom onset. CAGE 0/4.

Meds: None currently. Omeprazole—historic.

FamH: Noncontributory.

Physical Examination: Indicate only pertinent positive and negative findings related to the patient's chief complaint.

No physical exam.

Differential Diagnosis: In order of likelihood (with 1 being the most likely), list up to 5 potential or possible diagnoses for this patient's presentation (in many cases, fewer than 5 diagnoses are likely)	Diagnostic Work-up: List immediate plans (up to 5) for further diagnostic work-up
1. Peptic ulcer disease	1. CBC with differential
2. Acute gastritis	2. CXR, upright
3. Acute pancreatitis	3. CT scan, abdomen
4. Inflammatory bowel disease (Crohn's disease)	4. Liver function panel including: AST/ALT, bilirubin (fractionated), Amylase/lipase, alkaline phosphatase
5. Gallstone disease (cholecystitis, choledocholithiasis)	5. Basic metabolic profile including Ca.

37 Telephone Case: Elderly Fall

1. Opening Scenario

Marilyn O'Neal, the daughter of an 86-year-old female, has called the physician's office for advice about her mother's condition after a fall.

2. Vital Signs

Unreported

3. Examinee Tasks

1. Obtain a focused history.

2. Do not perform a physical examination and leave that portion blank on the patient note.

3. Discuss your initial diagnostic impression and your work-up plan.

4. After leaving the room, complete your patient note on the given form.

Introduce yourself, and place the first signpost.

"Hello, Ms. O'Neal, this is Dr. Pierce. How can I help you?"

"Hi Dr. Pierce. I'm calling because **my mom**, you know her, Lori? She **took a fall** this morning **when she came down the stairs**. I think she tumbled and went down the last few. I don't know that she fell all the way down but just the last ones."

"Oh, I'm sorry to hear that. Well, falls can be very dangerous, especially for the elderly. Please go on."

"**Sure**, she's alright now. She just seems like she took a tumble, but I know that can be a problem with old folks. She's 86 years old, you know."

"Yeah, it sure can. When did this happen?"

"Just a **few minutes ago**. Maybe, a **half-hour** or so. You see, she was coming down the stairs here, and I **heard her** fall on the bottom. I **didn't see it**. No one was around, but I heard her hit the ground. She was just laying there, so when I got to her she was **awake** and **picking herself up**, you know. I think she hurt her pride. Anyway, she said she **tripped on the last stair** and just went over. She said she didn't fall all the way from the top."

"Ok. Did she ever lose consciousness? Or was she unconscious when you found her?"

"**No**, no. At least not when I got there, and it was only a second later. I mean, she was awake but…she was maybe a **little dazed at first**. She

In an unwitnessed fall of an elderly, demented person, assume the worst-case scenario.

didn't remember it altogether at first. But then again, that just might be her **dementia**. That's why she lives with us, you know. She can't really live alone because she has dementia real bad. She **doesn't say much anyway**."

"Ok. Does it look like she hit her head at all?"

"**No**, it doesn't look like it. I'm looking now…**nothing that I can see**."

"Is she talking to you now?"

"**Yeah**, well sort of. **She's wondering who I am**. She started doing that **last week** for some reason. But, yeah, she's talking to me."

"Ok. I can imagine how hard that could be to try to tell a change. But, do you think she has had a change in her mental status since the fall?"

"I wish I could tell…**maybe**."

"Ok. I understand. Because it's so hard to tell, I'd first of all like you to make sure she is lying down on her back. Can you do that?"

First priority should be to ensure the patient's safety.

"**Yeah**. [in the background] The doctor says to lie down. On your back, mom. There you go."

"Ok, Marilyn? I'd also like you to make sure her back is straight. I'd like you to lay her on the ground if you can. But then try to take two pillows and just put them on both sides of her head, ok? So she can't turn her neck is what I'd like. Not under her head but on the sides to restrict her head movement."

"**Ok**, doctor. Hold on…Ok. She's on her back on the floor with the pillows."

"It can be very hard to keep her in a position like that. Do you think she will stay there?"

"**Yeah**, I told her to stay right there. My **husband** is also helping her."

"Ok, now. I'd like you to call an ambulance when we get off the phone, because the best way to get your mom checked out and transported safely is if it's done by professionals, ok?"

"**Ok**, I thought about that but wanted to call you first."

"I understand. It can be very hard to figure out what to do right away, especially if there doesn't seem to be anything wrong right away. Has your mother walked since the accident?"

"I **don't think so**. She just **crawled** to the couch sort of. **No**, she didn't actually walk."

Don't delay alerting EMS to the situation to obtain history.

"Ok. Sometimes when older folks fall, bones can be broken that aren't obvious at first. Just try to keep her still until an ambulance arrives, ok?"

"I'm having my husband call the ambulance on **his cell phone** right now so I can still be on the phone with you. He's calling right now."

"Ok. That's very good. I'll also call the emergency room and alert them to the accident. So I can do that, can I ask a few more questions about your mom?"

"**Sure**."

"*You said she had dementia. Has anyone told you a disease that might be causing that?*"

"They say it's because of **strokes** that keep happening to her. She **used to smoke** a long time, and so they did some brain scans on her, and they said she keeps having these strokes that affect her."

"*Ok. That's certainly a cause of dementia sometimes. Does your mom take any special medications for that?*"

"**Yeah**, they have her on one called **Coumadin** and some **aspirin** for it. That's supposed to prevent more of them."

"*Ok. Has she been taking her medicines regularly?*"

"**Yeah**, I give them to her so I know she is."

"*Is she on any other medicines?*"

"**Yeah**, she's on an inhaler called **advair** and one called **albuterol** when she needs it. She also has **oxygen** she uses at night and when we go outside the house."

"*Ok. Did she have the oxygen on when she fell?*"

"**No**, she didn't"

"*Ok. I'd like to ask you to go ahead and put the oxygen on her now, ok?*"

"**Ok**. I'll have my husband do it so we can talk. [in the background] Bill, put her oxygen on her, the doctor said."

"*That's good. Is she on any other medicines?*"

"Um, she also takes one called **alendronate** for her **bones**. She also takes a **multivitamin** and **calcium**, too."

"*Ok. Has she ever fallen before?*"

"**Not that we know of**. She hasn't had any types of falls."

"*How about any other medical problems?*"

"She has that **emphysema** from smoking all that time, then the **strokes**, and also **osteoporosis**—that's what that alendonate is for. Otherwise she's good."

"*Ok. Does she have any allergies to anything?*"

"**No**, nothing."

"*Has she ever had a surgery, especially one on any of her bones?*"

"**Nope**, nothing. Oh, doctor, I think the ambulance is here."

"*That's good, Marilyn. I'll let you go then and call the ER. I want you to tell the paramedics everything you can, ok?*"

"Ok, doctor. I'll tell them everything."

"*Ok. I'll be in contact with you after your mom gets seen at the ER, and I'll be involved in her case, ok? I'll let you go for now, though.*"

"Ok, doctor. They're here. I'll talk to you later. Bye."

"*Ok. Bye.*"

A fall for a patient on blood-thinning medication can be especially dangerous, not only for intracranial bleeding but also occult blood loss resulting from third spacing.

End of Case

PATIENT NOTE

History: Include significant positives and negatives from history of present illness, past medical history, review of system(s), social history, and family history.

HPI: Daughter of 86 y/o female s/p fall from stairs approximately ½-hour before phone call. Call was with daughter, Marilyn, who relayed history. Patient suffered unwitnessed fall down unknown number of stairs landing at the bottom. Pt has baseline dementia, including recall difficulty, but was found to be conscious and responsive seconds after the fall. Memory impaired to person. No obvious focal pain although pt did not ambulate. Upon instruction during call, daughter placed pt in supine position on floor with inline cervical stabilization using pillows. Ambulance called on another phone and did arrive during phone call. Call terminated when EMS arrived to residence for ease of daughter's interaction with EMS personnel.

Meds: Coumadin, aspirin, alendronate, advair, albuterol PRN, oxygen PRN.

PMH: Multi-infarct dementia, COPD, osteoporosis.

Smoking: Historic.

Physical Examination: Indicate only pertinent positive and negative findings related to the patient's chief complaint.

No physical exam.

Differential Diagnosis: In order of likelihood (with 1 being the most likely), list up to 5 potential or possible diagnoses for this patient's presentation (in many cases, fewer than 5 diagnoses are likely)	Diagnostic Work-up: List immediate plans (up to 5) for further diagnostic work-up.
1. Subdural hematoma	1. CT scan, head
2. Epidural hematoma	2. CT scan cervical spine.
3. Fracture	3. Plain X-rays—, chest, , bilateral hips, extremities as indicated
4. Cervical spine injury	4. CBC, Coagulation profile (pT, aPTT, INR)
5. Hemorrhagic stroke.	5. Electrolytes, renal function, and glucose

---

1. Opening Scenario

Clarice James, a 21-year-old G1P0 female, called the labor and delivery department stating she's having contractions.

2. Vital Signs

None reported

3. Examinee Tasks

1. Obtain a focused history.

2. Do not perform a physical examination and leave that portion blank on the patient note.

3. Discuss your initial diagnostic impression and your work-up plan.

4. After leaving the room, complete your patient note on the given form.
Press the speaker button on the phone to be connected with the caller.

Introduce yourself, and place the first signpost.

"Hello, Ms. James? I'm Dr. Feather. I'm the doctor on the labor and delivery floor this evening. What can I do for you?"

"Hi Dr. Feather, I'm pregnant and, well…really pregnant, and I want to know if I'm in **labor yet**. I don't know, and my doctor said to call this number if I had any questions about going into labor."

"That's a good idea. Sometimes it's hard to tell if you're in labor or not. Please let me get some information from you, and I can better understand the situation. Are you having any contractions or cramping?"

"Yeah, **I have cramps**, like, **every few minutes**. I slept last night with them, and I just figured it wasn't anything to worry about. That's why I'm calling. These **didn't go away**, and it feels weird."

"Contractions can feel differently in everyone, but they're generally low down in the pelvis and can feel somewhat like a menstrual type cramp or just pressure. Although, it's hard to say in each person. How do yours feel?"

"Kind of like **period cramps,** sort of. They weren't that bad, and I had some of this pain, sort of, during the pregnancy, but now it feels like period cramps. I don't want to come in over just cramps and you tell me I'm

> The distance from the hospital can be a clue to how aggressive to be with a patient's situation. If distance is a significant barrier, take the "better safe than sorry" approach.

worrying, though. I live about a **half-hour from the hospital,** and I don't want to drive that far if I'm just worrying for nothing, you know? But this is my **first baby**, so I don't know what to look for either."

"That's understandable. Are these feelings of cramps coming and going regularly?"

"**I guess so**. They started last night, and it was every now and then. Then all today they've gotten to be more and more frequent—maybe one every, like, **15 minutes** or something now."

"Ok. The best way to tell is for you to come in, and we'll evaluate you here. We have special tests we can run and ways to look at the activity your uterus might be having. These tests can tell us if you might be in labor. If you don't mind, may I ask a few more questions about your pregnancy?"

"**Yeah**, go ahead."

"How far along are you in your pregnancy? That is, do you know your due date?"

"It's not until **next month**. Like on the **15th**. I have one of those wheels here at the house and it says I'm **35 weeks and 4 days** along. That's why I didn't know if this was s'posed to happen."

"Well, that is a bit early. The possibility of having a baby early is another good reason to come in if you're in any doubt. That's because the new baby will probably need special care here in the hospital this early on. If you were to have it right now, the best chances of survival would be to have it here in the hospital. Have you had any vaginal discharge lately?"

"That's another thing, Dr. Feather. My doctor told me to expect some more discharge this late. I've had a bunch. But it's **not the regular**, you know, white stuff. It's **runny,** sort of."

"Would you say it was a watery-type discharge such as water from your tap, or is it still kind of thick?"

"It's **kind of like water**. At first, I thought "Geez, I'm peeing on myself," you know. But I don't know. I've gone through a bunch of underwear 'cause of it, and I'm trying not to pee."

"It does sound unusual. That's something else that's important to check when you get here. Sometimes the amniotic sac around the baby can rupture, or get a hole in it, too early. A little later in the pregnancy, many people describe their 'water breaking' as a sudden fluid leak, but sometimes a little hole can cause the fluid to leak out a little at a time. That can be a problem because that fluid can start early labor, or the hole might allow bacteria to get into the sac around the baby and cause an infection. I would recommend you come in soon to be checked. Can you do that?"

"**Sure**. I'll get some stuff together and come in now."

"Ok, just a few more questions so we can be ready for you when you get here. Have you had vaginal bleeding at all during this pregnancy?"

"**No**, not at all."

"Have you been able to feel the baby moving in the last few hours?"

"**Yeah**, it's a 'he.' He was moving a little bit ago."

Important information in this case:
  G's and P's
  Gestational age
  Contraction details
  Vaginal leakage
    details
  History of bleeding
  Baby movement
  Safe transport to the
    hospital

PROM can be a cause of preterm labor.

"Ok. Have you had regular doctor's appointments during this pregnancy?"

"**Yeah**, I was out of town for the last doctor's appointment but otherwise, yeah."

"Do you remember getting all your immunizations and tests done, especially in the beginning?"

"**Uh huh**. I got it all done."

"And were there any problems at all with any of the tests your doctor told you about?"

"**No**. He said I was good. I even **quit smoking** during this pregnancy."

"Well, that's great. Congratulations. How long ago did you quit?"

"About a **month** ago, I think. Finally did it though. I had been trying the whole time."

"Well, that's good. On a related point, have you had any alcohol during this pregnancy?"

"**No**, me and my husband were trying to get pregnant, so I haven't drank in a long time, 'cause we didn't know."

"Alright. Have you had a fever recently or even felt hot?"

"I **don't think so**. I haven't taken my temperature, but I don't feel like I'm hot."

"Ok. When was the last time you had sex?"

"A **couple of months**. My husband is in the Army, and he got deployed in May. He won't be back for a year or more. So, **I'm here without him**. That was the last time."

"Oh, I'm sorry to hear that. It's very hard when the father gets called up to serve before they get a chance to see their baby born. Do you have anyone there to help after the baby's born?"

"My **mom** was supposed to come down in about 2 weeks. She lives in Montana. She's not here now though. That's alright, my **best friend** can help **until mom gets here** if she needs to come."

"Ok. Can your friend drive you into the hospital tonight?"

"**Yeah**, she's here now so she knows what's going on."

"Ok. Our hospital also has social workers that can sometimes help in situations like these. They can help arrange community resources to make this time easier for you. We can talk more about that when you get here. In the meantime, are you allergic to any medicines?"

"**Nope**, nothing."

"Are you on any medications?"

"Just the **prenatal vitamins**, that's it."

"Ok. I'm going to let you go now so you can have your friend drive you in, ok? We'll make sure to be ready for you when you get here, ok? Do you have any questions for me?"

"I think we covered it. Do you think I'm in labor?"

"Well, it's hard to say without examining you ma'am. When you get here, I'll be able to do a good exam on you and also use an ultrasound machine to try to tell how much fluid is around the baby. We'll also place you on a uterine

Significant time smoking during the pregnancy still confers risk factors onto the fetus. Smoking is one risk factor of preterm labor.

If transport can't be assured with reliability, then an ambulance is a good choice.

monitor for a period of time to try to catch any contractions you might be having. I'd like to be able to tell you over the phone, but I can't. Listening to the situation, I'd highly recommend you come to the hospital right now so we can evaluate you. Do you think you can do that?"

"**Yeah**, I'm coming now."

"Ok. Please have your friend drive safely."

"Ok, bye."

"Bye."

End of Case

PATIENT NOTE

History: Include significant positives and negatives from history of present illness, past medical history, review of system(s), social history, and family history.

HPI: 21 y/o female G1P0 at reported 35 4/7 wks pregnancy with reported regular contractions and possible ROM. Contractions reported as q15 min. Denies vaginal bleeding. Reports positive fetal movement. History of smoking during pregnancy but denies alcohol use. OB history reported as regular visits without previous abnormality although she missed her last appointment. No reported fever or recent illness. Pt stated that a reliable friend would transport her which consisted of an approximately ½-hr ride to hospital. Father of baby (husband) unavailable for support because of military obligations.

Meds: Prenatal vitamins.

Physical Examination: Indicate only pertinent positive and negative findings related to the patient's chief complaint.

No physical exam.

Differential Diagnosis: In order of likelihood (with 1 being the most likely), list up to 5 potential or possible diagnoses for this patient's presentation (in many cases, fewer than 5 diagnoses are likely)	Diagnostic Work-up: List immediate plans (up to 5) for further diagnostic work-up
1. Preterm rupture of membranes	1. Sterile speculum exam (evaluate for pooling of amniotic fluid, ferning of discharge by microscopy, and nitrizine testing of discharge)
2. Prolonged rupture of membranes	2. Amniotic fluid index (ultrasound)
3. Preterm labor	3. Cervical exam
4. Braxton-Hicks (false labor) contractions	4. Nonstress test (Recording uterine activity and fetal heart rate for 20 min)
5. Cervical or vaginal infection	5.

39   Telephone Case: Question of Abuse

---

1. Opening Scenario

Kelly Richards has called your physician's clinic about her daughter, Joey, a 3-year-old female, regarding possible abuse.

2. Vital Signs

Unreported

3. Examinee Tasks

1. Obtain a focused history.

2. Do not perform a physical examination and leave that portion blank on the patient note.

3. Discuss your initial diagnostic impression and your work-up plan.

4. After leaving the room, complete your patient note on the given form.
Press the speaker button on the telephone to be connected to the caller.

Introduce yourself, and place the first signpost.

"Hi, Ms. Richards? It's Dr. Humboldt. What can I help you with today?"

"Hi, doctor. I…I have a question. I mean you probably get questions all the time, but I have a question **about my daughter**."

"Ok. Please go ahead."

"Well, I'm wondering…I mean, I'm wondering what **abuse** might look like on a **3-year-old**? I mean, I've seen some marks on my baby girl, and I don't know but I just don't know what they're from."

"Do you mean sexual abuse or marks that she might get from physical abuse?"

"I mean the **sexual** kind. I mean…she just isn't acting like herself when I change her. And she's really **irritable** for no reason lately, and then I saw all these marks on her. I mean, what's it look like? If I were to think, you know, if someone was doing something to her?"

"Well, sexual abuse is very hard to tell on one aspect alone, ma'am. Sexual abuse especially might cause small cuts on the genitals or rashes or just redness or swelling. Commonly, there is no outward appearance at all. I'm sorry to hear this might be going on. It's a very difficult thing to confront, but I'd like to examine Joey in the office to better evaluate any possible problems."

"Do you think it would look like cuts and welts?"

> Don't commit to specifying a certain appearance of abuse because it can look so different in each case. Keep the description broad and stress expert examination.

Consider the two agendas:
Patient's agenda—To obtain an answer or clues to be able to determine if abuse is present.
Physician's agenda—To persuade the caller to bring in the child for determination of abuse.

"*It's very hard to tell in each instance, Ms. Richards. Abuse is a matter that isn't solely determined based on the finding of any one sign. Abuse can come in so many forms that there are a lot of different appearances. I think it's best if you come in and we can properly address everything that might be going on. We have a social worker who is a counselor who can also talk with you about the situation and help determine if abuse is likely. She can also talk with Joey and work out the situation. Do you think you could come in for me?*"

"I mean…I don't want to make a big deal out of it. I'm probably crazy. I don't want to start something and do something bad for no reason. I mean…I don't know. I just don't know. I'm going to just think about it for awhile."

"*Well, of course you can think about it for awhile. But I also don't want you to make a decision to not be evaluated and be wondering if there is something that can be done or not. Please keep in mind, coming in to the office would absolutely not be accusing anyone of anything. In fact, being evaluated by us wouldn't necessarily lead to any actions at all. When you get here, we can have our social worker talk with you and Joey, and if there's a reason for concern, she may also involve the department called Child Protective Services. However, when you come here, we will offer you resources and a safe haven so you can do what's best for you and your child. Keep in mind, we need to get Joey the help she needs and that may be through the use of our resources here.*"

"What would you do?"

"*Well, when you get here, we'd talk with you about the situation and have you explain exactly what might be going on, and then we'd do an exam on Joey, with you present, to determine if there are any marks that might have been caused by something like abuse. We would also take samples of fluid and photographs to test for things we can't see. Most of all, though, we'd provide a safe environment for you to talk about the situation and make sure you're in a safe place.*"

"I know…I…this is horrible, but I just don't want to hurt anyone. I'm scared about this but I'm not going to accuse…anyone of this kind of thing, you know. I mean, I don't know."

"*I understand that, ma'am. I'd like to provide you with the best answers I can and do what's best for Joey in every aspect. The last thing I, or any of us here at the clinic, want to do is break up a family. On the other hand, ma'am, the best way to protect children is to make sure people who cause them harm don't have contact with them. I can't guarantee an agency such as Child Welfare and Protective Services won't need to be involved, but if they do, I firmly believe it would be best for Joey and yourself.*"

"Yeah."

"*Can I ask a few questions of you?*"

"Yeah."

"*How old is Joey?*"

"She's **3 years old**."

"*What do the marks look like?*"

"They're on her **privates** and look like **red marks** sort of. Kind of like a **skinned knee** down there. But she also looks, like, **swollen**. And she cries when I wipe her there. She looks really painful."

Reaching out for help during a time of suspected abuse leaves the caregiver feeling very vulnerable and in need of much assurance. Demonstrate your willingness to listen and empathize over the phone to assure her that's what she'll find upon arrival.

"Ok. How long has she acted like this and had these marks?"

"I just **noticed** it **last night**. She came back from her **dad's** last night. He had both of the kids **over the weekend**. He takes them all the time, and this is the first time anything like this has ever happened."

"Ok. Does she have a negative reaction to anyone she comes in contact with?"

"**No**, when he dropped her off she was fine. She didn't cry, she was fine."

"Since you have had her back, has she had any problems toileting?"

"**Yeah**, she doesn't want to go. She is, like, **shy** about it. I have her in those pull up pants, you know, because she's kind of slow to potty train. And she **doesn't want me changing her now**. I mean, that's **new**, you know."

"Ok. Has that only been the last day or has that been longer?"

"Well, maybe **last week** too, a little, but more since she came back. **I work the weekends** so I can't have her all the time. I have to drop her off. I mean, **what am I supposed to do?**"

"Ma'am, I can't say there's anything going on over the phone at all. Sometimes it's hard because you might have those job and money pressures. I can't say I have the answer, either. I just think if the abuse is suspected, it's most important to make sure the baby's safe. She really needs to be evaluated here, and we can help sort the situation out."

"Ok. So if I come in, you say I'm not going to have to do anything? I mean, **I'm not coming in if you say you are going to take my baby away from me**."

"I certainly can't say what will happen if we determine Joey has had an incidence of abuse. That is, that's just out of my hands, but I can tell you it's also not up to me. I'd like to tell you the Child Protective Services and our social worker will make the determination of what to do. However, keep in mind, they certainly have no interest in accusing anyone of abuse or taking children. If it's determined there may be abuse going on, they will certainly help you in any way they can. If that includes giving you and Joey a safe place to stay for some time, then that's what they'll do. If at all possible, these agencies don't want to see the child separated from the parents at all. The best thing for you to do in the situation you're in, for both yourself and Joey, is to be seen by the people who work with this commonly, ok?"

"Well…**ok**."

"Do you feel safe right now? That is, do you think anyone in your household would hurt you if you came in?"

"**Yeah**. I mean, I don't feel like I'm going to be beaten or anything."

"Ok. You also mentioned you have another child there. When you come in, can you bring them, too?"

"**Yeah**, that's my **8-year-old**. He's at the neighbor's right now, but I can get him."

"Ok. Is there any reason to think he might have been involved in this as well?"

"**No**, I…I don't think so. I'm just scared."

"I can understand that, Ms. Richards. Remember, we're just trying to help the best way possible. There's no fingers being pointed at all right now."

Newly developed toileting issues can be a behavior pattern consistent with abuse.

Financial pressures are a major risk factor in abusive situations.

The mother is constantly looking for answers to her agenda: Can I use any tidbits the doctor says to judge for myself if there's abuse? It's important to keep reinforcing your agenda to have her come to the clinic.

"Ok. **I just don't know if anything's going on, and I want to make sure she's safe**."

"That's your job as a mom, I think. I think you're doing nothing but the best thing for your kids. Your job as a parent is to protect your kids. That's the right thing to do."

"**Yeah**."

"Ok. Can I expect you to come in today, then?"

"**Yeah**, I can come in."

"Ok. We'll wait for you then. Ok?"

"Alright, Dr Humboldt. **I'll be there shortly**."

"Ok. Bye."

"Bye."

End of Case

PATENT NOTE

PATIENT NOTE

History: Include significant positives and negatives from history of present illness, past medical history, review of system(s), social history, and family history.

HPI: Telephone call from mother of a 3 y/o female with newly discovered genital lesions suspected to be c/w sexual abuse. Mother states marks are on child's genital region and include welt like appearance and swelling. Child has also acted fussy x 1 week and has had some toileting irritability during this time. Custody shared between separated parents with discovery of these markings upon return of child from weekend visitation with father. Mother tearful on interview but agreed to presentation to clinic on same day as call.

Physical Examination: Indicate only pertinent positive and negative findings related to the patient's chief complaint.

No physical exam.

Differential Diagnosis: In order of likelihood (with 1 being the most likely), list up to 5 potential or possible diagnoses for this patient's presentation (in many cases, fewer than 5 diagnoses are likely)	Diagnostic Work-up: List immediate plans (up to 5) for further diagnostic work-up
1. Sexual abuse	1. Urinanalysis and urine culture
2. Physical abuse	2. Vaginal, oral, and anal microscopic slides and culture performed
3. Accidental trauma	3. Gonorrhea and Chlamydia antigen testing on genital and oral samples
4. Urinary tract infection	4. RPR, HIV antibodies, hepatitis B and C testing
5. Candidiasis	5. Hair and nail samples

1. Opening Scenario

JoAnn Johnson has called your emergency department about her son, Caleb Johnson, a 6-year-old male, who has reportedly ingested cleaning chemicals.

2. Vital Signs

Unreported

3. Examinee Tasks

1. Obtain a focused history.

2. Do not perform a physical examination and leave that portion blank on the patient note.

3. Discuss your initial diagnostic impression and your work-up plan.

4. After leaving the room, complete your patient note on the given form.
Press the speaker button on the telephone to be connected to the caller.

Introduce yourself, and place the first signpost.

"Hello, Ms. Johnson? This is Dr. Smith. I understand your son has gotten into some chemicals at home. Can you tell me more about this, please?"

"Yes, doctor. Thank you so much for calling me back so quickly. I'm beside myself with worry. Caleb, he's **6 years old**, was playing in the kitchen. I had to go to my bedroom to shut off the television and make the bed, and when I came back, he was crying and sitting **under the sink** in the cabinet. I could hear him, he was hiding from me. I opened the cupboard and he was there amongst all my cleaning supplies crying. He had **thrown up some green fluid**. He looked at me and **said he drank some** and it hurts. I grabbed him and **called right away**."

"Ok. Please calm down, we're going to work through this and then talk about what to do, ok? How long ago do you think he drank the chemical?"

"It was only about **5 or 10 minutes ago**."

"Do you have any idea what it was?"

"I think it was the **drain cleaner**. All the cleaners and stuff are knocked over, but he was closest to the drain cleaner. It's also a **green color, and his lips** look a little green and **so does what he threw up**."

> When talking to an excited parent, be as confident and reassuring as possible. Your calm may be the only calm there is.

"Ok. Can you look at the drain cleaner and tell me what it says the 'active ingredient' is?"

"Yes, I've got it right here. Do you think he'll be alright?"

"I think he'll be fine, ma'am. I need you to make sure you're calm, and we'll find out what happened."

"Ok. It says it's **potassium hydroxide**. I don't know what that is."

"Ok. That's a special type of chemical used in those types of products. Can you gather all the other chemicals under the sink and tell me what they are?"

"Yes, I'm looking…It looks like there's some **soap**. The **liquid** kind and some **dry** kind. The liquid kind is open. And some **glass cleaner**. That's all that's down here except other brillo pads."

"Ok. Now, if that's all that's there, it sounds like the worst thing is the drain cleaner. Does he still have some green on his lips?"

"**No**, he's crying and my husband has him. He's **drooling** a lot and **won't stop crying**."

"Alright. Is he acting unusual in any other way? Such as vomiting?"

"**Yeah**, he's **vomited twice** since this. My husband has him in the bathroom but I know he's vomited twice."

"Is he breathing ok, or is he struggling to get air in?"

"**No**, he's just crying. He's **coughing** a lot too. My husband said he vomited up more of that green liquid. It looks just like the **drain cleaner**."

"Alright, ma'am. Is he breathing fast or about the same as when he normally cries?"

"**No**, he's breathing ok."

"Are there any unusual noises when he breathes? Such as a high-pitched sound called wheezing?"

"**No**, he's alright. It just looks like he's in pain."

"I can imagine. Ms. Johnson, I want you to bring Caleb to the hospital. Do you have a car?"

"**Yes**, yes, we can bring him in."

"Before you go, I want to have you gather everything from under the sink where you found Caleb. Please take everything, even those items you don't think he ingested."

"**Ok**. I can do that."

"Also, please bring any medications Caleb may be taking. Anything he might have taken in the last few days."

"Ok. He's on his medicine for **ADHD**. I'll bring that too."

"Does Caleb have any other medical problems?"

"He has **ADHD**. Nothing else."

"Ok. How far from the hospital are you now?"

"We live just down the street. About **10 minutes**. I'm talking on a cell phone so I can keep talking, too."

Potassium hydroxide is a common chemical classified as a strong alkali. This gives a clue to the fact that a caustic agent which may induce alkali burns may be at work.

Assess the best and fastest way of transport in a situation where a caustic agent and possible aspiration are present. If the parents are capable, that is likely the fastest way.

"Ms. Johnson, I want to let you go so you aren't talking on the phone and driving at the same time. I know this is a very stressful time, and I don't want you to be distracted by talking to me. I have enough information that we'll know what to do with him here. I just want you to concentrate on driving here safely, ok?"

"Ok."

"When you get to the hospital, drive right into the emergency entrance, and we'll be able to take care of you the fastest."

"Ok. We'll leave now."

"Ok, Ms. Johnson. We'll be prepared to take care of Caleb as soon as you get here. Be very careful on the drive over, ok? We'll see you in a few minutes."

"Ok doctor. Goodbye."

Make sure the excited parent isn't distracted from driving while talking on the phone. Staying on the phone with you won't improve the prognosis but may cause a motor vehicle accident.

End of Case

PATIENT NOTE

History: Include significant positives and negatives from history of present illness, past medical history, review of system(s), social history, and family history.

HPI: 6 y/o male with reported ingestion of potassium hydroxide-containing drain cleaner. Ingestion approx 10 minutes before contact by phone. Co-ingestions reported as detergents and window cleaner, although all agents unverified. Pt witnessed to have drain cleaner on lips and in vomitis. Current symptoms reported as vomiting, drooling, cough, and uncontrollable crying.

PMH: ADHD.

Meds: Unknown ADHD medication.

Physical Examination: Indicate only pertinent positive and negative findings related to the patient's chief complaint.

No physical exam.

Differential Diagnosis: In order of likelihood (with 1 being the most likely), list up to 5 potential or possible diagnoses for this patient's presentation (in many cases, fewer than 5 diagnoses are likely)	Diagnostic Work-up: List immediate plans (up to 5) for further diagnostic work-up
1. Caustic alkali ingestion	1. Arterial blood gas
2. Detergent ingestion	2. Electrolytes and renal function
3. Orophayrngeal and esophageal injury	3. CXR, upright, PA/Lat
4. Aspiration	4. CBC
5. Gastrointestinal perforation	5.

Index

Note: Page numbers followed by *f* and *t* denote figures and tables, respectively.